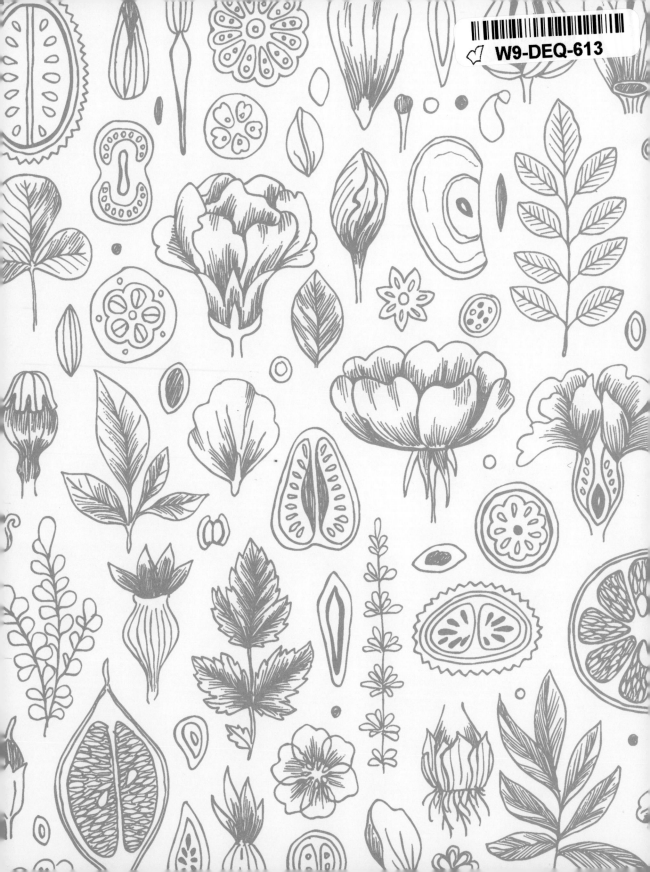

Peaceful Kitchen

Peaceful Kitchen

MORE THAN 100 COZY PLANT-BASED
RECIPES TO COMFORT
THE BODY AND NOURISH THE SOUL

Catherine Perez, RD

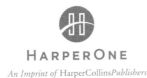

HarperOne

An Imprint of HarperCollins*Publishers*

HarperCollins books may be purchased for educational, business, or sales promotional use. For information, please email the Special Markets Department at SPsales@harpercollins.com.

FIRST EDITION

Designed by Elina Cohen

Unless otherwise noted, photographs are provided by the author
Photograph on p. xiv by Shelly Xu

Illustrations courtesy of Shutterstock: florals © Kate Macate; borders © MarinaStorm; part watercolor © KatMoys; mango © Rina Oshi; botanicals © adehoidar; nutritional label © BROTH; watercolor mango © Lyubov Tolstova; cinnamon, cardamom, black peppercorns, and vanilla pods © Net Vector; raspberry © DiViArt ; radish, onion, pepitas, kabocha squash, ginger, bell pepper, carrot, tomato, and jalapeno © Svesla Tasla; watercolor kale, watercolor garlic, and watercolor carrot © Katflare; cilantro, dill, and coriander seeds © QualityDesigner; corn, garlic, cabbage, onion, and scallions © Nikiparonak; watercolor avocado, watercolor lemon, and serrano © vasabii; shitake mushroom © Sketch Master; sweet potato © Epine; watercolor chickpeas © Daria Ustiugova; lime and lemon © SpicyTruffel; pepitas © QualitDesigner

Library of Congress Cataloging-in-Publication Data has been applied for.

ISBN 978-0-06-332257-8

24 25 26 27 28 LBC 5 4 3 2 1

To my husband, Gregory. Thank you for always believing in me even when I don't. The impossible always seems way more manageable when I have you in my corner.

And to you, my community. To every one of you who have followed along in this journey, for every message of encouragement and every click you made to my website, thank you! I can't ever express how much you mean to me and how you gave me the opportunity to pursue a career I absolutely love. I hope that this book gives you as much love and comfort as you have provided to me.

Contents

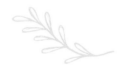

CHAPTER 1. BREAKING THE FAST

CHAPTER 2. SATISFYING SALADS

CHAPTER 3. GRAB IT & GO

CHAPTER 4. NOURISHING BOWLS

CHAPTER 5. NUTRIENT-PACKED MAINS

CHAPTER 6. ELEVATED VEGGIES

CHAPTER 7. SNACKS & SWEETS

CHAPTER 8. SAUCEOLOGY

Introduction

In some ways, I find the title *Peaceful Kitchen* kind of ironic because the kitchen wasn't always a peaceful place for me. It started out more chaotic. And by chaotic, I mean almost burning down the kitchen on multiple occasions. So it's a miracle that I've found myself talking to the world about food, let alone sharing it with you. For me, as for so many, food has been a joyful, challenging, educational, transformative journey. So let's start at the beginning.

When I was growing up, I wanted nothing to do with cooking. In fact, I remember a conversation with my Dominican mother, who shared her concern that I didn't have any strong cooking or cleaning skills under my belt for my future husband. I would say, "I'll just marry someone who will do that for me." Why not? My mom already cooked delicious Dominican food that included guisado (stewed meats), Moro, plátanos fritos (fried plantains), and habichuelas (stewed beans), all served with a side of steamed frozen veggies. We also had plenty of the standard grocery essentials at home—all kinds of snacks, cookies, and frozen pizzas stocked and ready to keep me "alive." As far as I was concerned, I was set, and I would simply eat what I wanted and what was available to me. Why learn to cook?

Over the years, I developed a major sweet tooth. I was particularly enamored by cookies. If there was a bag of them in the pantry, those cookies would not survive the evening. I also loved to add sugar to everything. Think four tablespoons of sugar over cornflakes for breakfast, and when the adults were having coffee, I was adding a few tablespoons of sugar to my black tea, too. At the same time, I was constantly asking my mom for fried foods like plátanos con salchichón (fried plantains and salami) or asking for money to go to Burger King for a fried chicken club sandwich.

I was happy with my eating habits, or at least, I thought I was. I never truly reflected on what I was putting in my body until someone I cared about was diagnosed with prediabetes and high cholesterol. When they came home with all the paperwork from their doctor, we read over a list of foods to avoid.

"So what do I eat, then?" I didn't have an answer for them at the time. I didn't even know that food would be involved in the discussion.

"I don't know, but I'll find out."

I started researching, and after weeding through a lot of harmful health information available at the time (some things just never change), we worked on managing their symptoms and trying to make better food choices available at home when we could. And of course, the more I learned, the more concerned I became about my own health. Slowly, I began making changes to the way I ate. Were those changes perfectly executed? Absolutely not. I made my fair share of mistakes and fell into a lot of diet traps. I counted calories, reduced my carbs, and even tried to exercise excessively. All of it just didn't feel good, and it didn't feel right. Luckily, I have learned from my mistakes and used my biology degree to do better research.

The more I dove into nutrition research, the more I wanted to learn. I wanted to know about all the nutrients in specific foods and loved reading about the ways people of different cultures ate and how that impacted their overall health. Eventually, I stumbled across some research and information regarding plant-based eating and veganism. I was intrigued, but I kept thinking that there was no way I could make that big of a change. Regardless, I kept coming back to the idea of it because it felt so aligned with all my "whys." At the heart of it all, I wanted to:

EAT MORE PLANTS TO HELP SUPPORT MY HEALTH GOALS
AND TAKE PREVENTATIVE ACTIONS EARLY;

REDUCE HARM TO ANIMALS (INCLUDING PEOPLE),
ESPECIALLY AFTER LEARNING SO MUCH ABOUT HOW MY FOOD
GOT TO MY PLATE; AND

TREAD LIGHTLY ON THE EARTH, REDUCING MY IMPACT ON CLIMATE
CHANGE AND DOING MY PART TO PROTECT THE ENVIRONMENT.

All of it just made so much sense to me, so one day back in 2009, I went vegan cold ~~turkey~~ tofu. Now, let's not forget that I was a disaster in the kitchen *and* that I have a Dominican mother. When I told my mom that I wasn't eating meat anymore, let alone any animal products, she was a bit hurt, confused, and angry. She told me that I would need to figure it out on my own. So I finally had to learn to cook for myself.

I printed out online recipes, watched a lot of Food Network to learn some basic techniques, and purchased my own cutting board and knife. With a lot of trial and error, I started learning the basics of cooking and making edible food. This process alone made me even more passionate about food and nutrition. Eventually, that "edible food" became even better as I experimented with different seasonings and cooking techniques. Then I started watching my mom cook and finding ways to keep my culture in my food and in my life. I felt so empowered.

With all that I learned, I desperately wanted to share and educate. I was feeling good and nourished, my blood work was looking so much better than it used to, and I felt like I was making a positive impact. I became so passionate about what I was doing to the point I wanted to make a full career change and become a dietitian. So I did!

I knew I wanted to focus my career around prevention in the realm of health and wellness and thought at most I would be a dietitian who counseled patients one-on-one. I would have loved that, but I still loved cooking and wanted it to be part of my work. Honestly, it's one thing to tell someone you should try adding some fruits and vegetables to a meal, but it's a completely different act to show someone how to do that and make it enjoyable. So I started sharing more of my own recipe ideas with my clients in sessions, and then started sharing the recipes on social media as a fun hobby. I could not have predicted the incredible community that has gathered around me as I have grown into being the Plant-Based RD.

This "hobby" had me spending way more time in the kitchen, but each time I was there, I felt comforted, at peace. Chopping became therapeutic, and plating all the food became an artistic escape. Through the creation and enjoyment of nourishing foods, I found deep solace. The kitchen that once gave me a lot of grief quickly became a place of comfort and escape. I want that same peace for you. In the following pages, we will explore a delicious array of ingredients, techniques, and recipes that will foster your own sense of peace and well-being in the kitchen.

So welcome. Have a seat at the table; I have so much to share with you.

XO Catherine

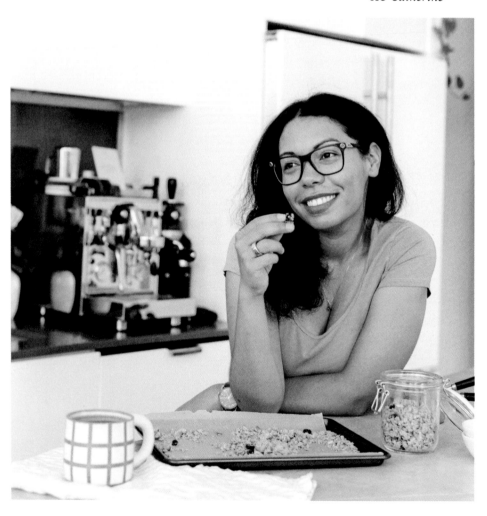

My Food Philosophy

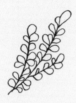

My life as a vegan dietitian has been a whirlwind at best, and despite the title, I don't go around slapping doughnuts out of people's hands, and I don't tell people what to eat. I also don't shame people for their food choices, even when they aren't aligned with my own professional advice. I always try to remember that once upon a time, I didn't know what I know now. Not to mention, change isn't always easy, even when you have the information in front of you. What I care most about is your story and how together we can help you build a better relationship with food without the fearmongering. Instead, I'll share evidence-based nutrition information while also showing you how to apply it to the plates you eat from daily. Then, it's up to you to do with that information as you please.

At the end of the day, this book is meant as a safe space for people to explore all things veganism and plant-forward eating. Regardless of how you eat, we can all benefit from adding more plants to our plates, which in turn helps support the health of us, the animals, and the planet.

WHAT IS THE DIFFERENCE BETWEEN VEGAN AND PLANT-BASED?

Veganism at its core is an ethical choice, not a diet. Veganism seeks to exclude all forms of cruelty toward animals to the best of your ability. As a result, vegans avoid the consumption of all animal-derived products, including meat, poultry, seafood, dairy, eggs, and honey. It's also important to note that veganism extends beyond one's food choices and focuses on lifestyle choices as well. This may include animal and human activism and choosing clothing and cosmetics that don't contain animal derived or tested ingredients.

A plant-based diet speaks specifically to how one eats. Typically, this approach of eating focuses on health and wellness with an emphasis on consuming primarily whole, unprocessed plant foods without negative ethical connotations attached. Vegans can consume a plant-based diet, but you don't have to be vegan to benefit from plant-based dietary choices.

I am vegan and work to continue minimizing harm where I can. I am comfortable in this choice. Ultimately, it's up to you how you wish to identify. I say this without judgment. Any work toward vegan or more plant-based eating leads to a reduction of harm, and it's never too late to start making changes. Something is always better than nothing! We do so much better when we think of what we can do instead of what we can't do. So even if you are not ready to commit 100 percent, consider that the small things you do can have a huge impact and more closely align your actions with your morals. At the end of the day, there is no such thing as a perfect vegan, but we can do our best each day to live with our best intentions.

BEFORE YOU GET STARTED

Let's internalize a few things before you decide to make any changes.

FOOD IS NOURISHMENT

It's very easy to start thinking about food in terms of numbers, but I encourage you to really look at your food as an opportunity to nourish yourself. When you nourish yourself to meet your specific needs, you'll feel good and want to continue eating the foods that make you feel your best. So put the focus on counting the types and number of plants you're eating instead of the calories.

GO AT YOUR OWN PACE

Not everyone can make a 100 percent shift in their lifestyle overnight. Both your body and your mind need time to get used to changes, and that's totally acceptable. In my own practice, I find that those who take this journey one step at a time learn better and set up more realistic expectations for themselves along the way. Start with small adjustments like making a conscious effort to add a vegetable to your dinner plate or replacing some of the meat on your plate with some well-seasoned lentils. When you're ready, continue working your way up. Try a meatless Monday or plan a few plant-based lunches during the week.

ADD, DON'T SUBTRACT

When it comes to making a dietary change, it's very easy to think of what you aren't "allowed" to eat. I like to frame it differently and put the focus on all the things you can add. It makes room for trying new foods, new cooking techniques, and new flavors that you may end up loving even more than the food you've always eaten.

MAKE APPROPRIATE SWAPS

Don't just take animal products off your plate and call it a day. Make an appropriate swap to replace it. For example, while I love mushroom tacos, mushrooms are not an adequate protein replacement for meat on their own. A more protein-rich option might be adding beans to it or some shredded tofu. This concept can also be applied to food experiences. If the thought of giving up something you love bothers you, find an alternative to it that fits. If you're an ice cream lover, try a dairy-free alternative. Love, cookies? Try making some vegan cookies yourself or buying them. And if ultimately you are not ready to make a swap, refocus on a different food you are more ready and able to change. Can't give up cheese? That's okay. Maybe swapping your milk for a plant-based alternative is easier. Go with that instead.

PERSONALIZE

There is no one-size-fits-all method to eating plant-based. Everyone has their own specific nutrient needs that can change based on age, height, weight, activity level, muscle mass, and disease states. We also have our own specific food preferences. There may be foods or flavors that you prefer over others. Knowing what you like will make this journey so much more enjoyable.

STAY TRUE TO YOURSELF

I thought for a long time that going vegan would mean that I could no longer partake in my favorite cultural foods. Spoiler alert: that wasn't the case. If anything, I feel more connected with my culture now. I was so eager to learn the traditional way of making a dish so that I could conceptualize making the most authentic plant-based version of it I could. Embracing my culture has only made this lifestyle stick.

STRIVE FOR PROGRESS

We are human. We are not designed to be perfect. You will make mistakes on your journey, and you'll probably feel bad about them. I know I have in the past! You might miss an ingredient on a label or be accidentally "dairy-ed" when you order a coffee out. I promise, it's okay and it's not worth agonizing over. Acknowledge it, see what you can do to avoid it from happening again, and just keep moving forward.

Plant-Based Nutrition Basics

According to the Academy of Nutrition and Dietetics, an appropriately planned vegetarian, vegan, or plant-based diet is "healthful, nutritionally adequate, and may provide health benefits for the prevention and treatment of certain diseases."*

When you are eating more vegetables, fruits, legumes, soy foods, whole grains, nuts, and seeds, you are consuming foods that tend to be lower in saturated fat and rich in fiber and antioxidants. Dietary patterns like this may help with lowering cholesterol and blood glucose levels, which contribute to a lower risk of developing: heart disease, type 2 diabetes, hypertension, and certain types of cancers.

---

* Vesanto Melina, Winston Craig, and Susan Levin, "Position of the Academy of Nutrition and Dietetics: Vegetarian Diets," *Journal of the Academy of Nutrition and Dietetics* 116, no. 12 (2016): 1970–80, https://doi.org/10.1016/j.jand.2016.09.025.

LET'S LOOK AT THE BIG PICTURE

You aren't going to wither away on a properly planned plant-based diet. In fact, you can thrive following this lifestyle. To do that, we need to make sure we understand some basics and acknowledge that there are certain nutrients we need to pay closer attention to. A good way to visualize what to prioritize is by comparing it to our typical plates.

The goal of this visual is to help identify the nutrient-dense food groups we should be including *most of the time* at each meal and realistically fill in the gaps as needed with other foods and supplements. With that said, this plate is also flexible because everyone's needs, cultural practices, and food access are unique. Some people will need more of a specific nutrient or food group for various reasons, and there is nothing wrong with that. If you are unsure of how to adjust portions or just want to make sure you are appropriately meeting your needs, meet with a dietitian to tailor amounts as needed.

This plate is not meant to be absolute. There are going to be times when you can't get a certain food group in. Realistically, some meals just won't fit these guidelines, and that is completely okay. When it comes to nutrition, the thing that will have the biggest impact on your health and well-being is what you are doing most of the time.

WHAT YOU CAN START ADDING TO YOUR PLATE

FRUITS AND VEGETABLES

The goal is to aim to fill half your plate with produce, and there's no secret as to why. Fruits and vegetables provide a wide array of vitamins, minerals, fiber, and antioxidants that can help reduce the risk of developing chronic disease.

It's important to eat plenty of fruits and veggies with a focus on varying your choices. An easy way to achieve this is by focusing on eating from a range of different colored fruits and veggies. For example, green cruciferous veggies, such as kale, bok choy, and broccoli, can provide an excellent source of calcium to help support bone health. Then you have yellow and orange veggies, such as carrots, butternut squash, and bell peppers, that will help you meet your vitamin A needs, which plays a role in normal immune function and eye health.

Using this method can help with getting you closer to the five daily servings of fruit

THE PLANT PLATE METHOD

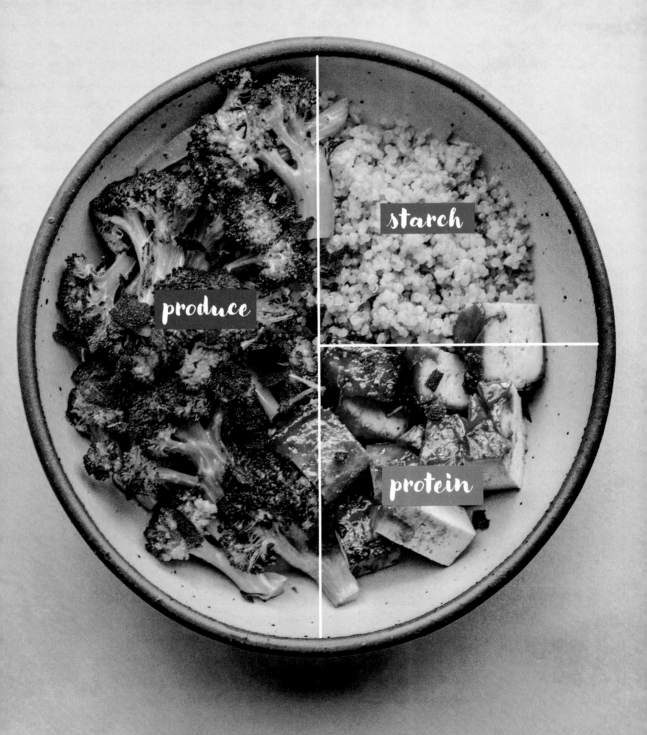

and veggies recommended to maintain long-term health.* Regardless, any intentional addition of produce can still lead to better health outcomes.

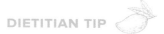

DIETITIAN TIP

Frozen and canned fruits and vegetables count! These options tend to be more affordable and won't go bad as quickly as fresh produce will. Be mindful of added sodium and added sugars. For canned fruit, choose options that are packed in 100 percent juice. If it's available, try low-sodium or no-salt-added canned vegetables or rinse them well using a colander under running water to help remove a significant amount of the sodium.

STARCHES AND GRAINS

Carbs are important. There, I said it! That's why you see that they are included on this plate and take up a quarter of it. We've all heard how carbs are detrimental to our health, how we can see shrinking numbers on the scale if we cut them out of our diet, but carbs provide essential nutrients we need.

Let's start viewing carbohydrates for what they are: a source of energy to fuel us; vitamins, minerals, and antioxidants to protect us; and fiber to help us stay regulated. Want the most benefit? Focus on consuming complex carbohydrates, like starchy vegetables and whole grains, as they are loaded with these nutrients. Consuming more whole grains and fiber may help to reduce cardiovascular disease risk and improve blood glucose control—not to mention feed the good bacteria in our gut to better support and regulate digestion.

Choose the carbohydrates you love. For some examples of complex carbohydrates, try oatmeal, whole grain rice, whole grain breads, wheat or corn tortillas, whole grain pastas, quinoa, farro, barley, millet, teff, amaranth, buckwheat, sweet potatoes, white potatoes, corn, and so much more.

---

* Dong D. Wang, Yanping Li, Shilpa N. Bhupathiraju, et al., "Fruit and Vegetable Intake and Mortality: Results From 2 Prospective Cohort Studies of US Men and Women and a Meta-Analysis of 26 Cohort Studies," *Circulation* 143, no. 17 (April 2021): 1642–54, https://doi.org/10.1161/CIRCULATIONAHA.120.048996.

If you are not a fan of brown rice, it's okay to eat white rice. Just make sure to incorporate whole grains elsewhere. The goal is to make at least half of the daily servings of grain you eat come from whole grains for the increased fiber benefit! The exact amount you need will vary depending on your specific nutrient needs.

PLANT-BASED PROTEINS

While you can absolutely meet your protein needs on a plant-based diet, don't take this nutrient lightly. While severe protein deficiencies are very rare in the general population, it is still possible to fall short on what you need. Not eating enough protein can make you feel fatigued and weak. On top of that, you need enough protein to help maintain adequate muscle mass, maintain bone health, and support immune function.

One of the easiest ways to make sure you are consuming enough protein is to aim for at least three or more servings of legumes daily. These include beans, chickpeas, peas, lentils, soy foods (tofu, tempeh, edamame, and TVP), and peanuts. Other protein-containing options include seitan, quinoa, and most vegan meat replacements.

PROTEIN SOURCE	SERVING AMOUNT
Beans or lentils, cooked	½ cup
Peanut butter	2 tablespoons
Peanuts	¼ cup
Soy milk or pea protein milk	1 cup
Tofu, tempeh, or TVP	½ cup

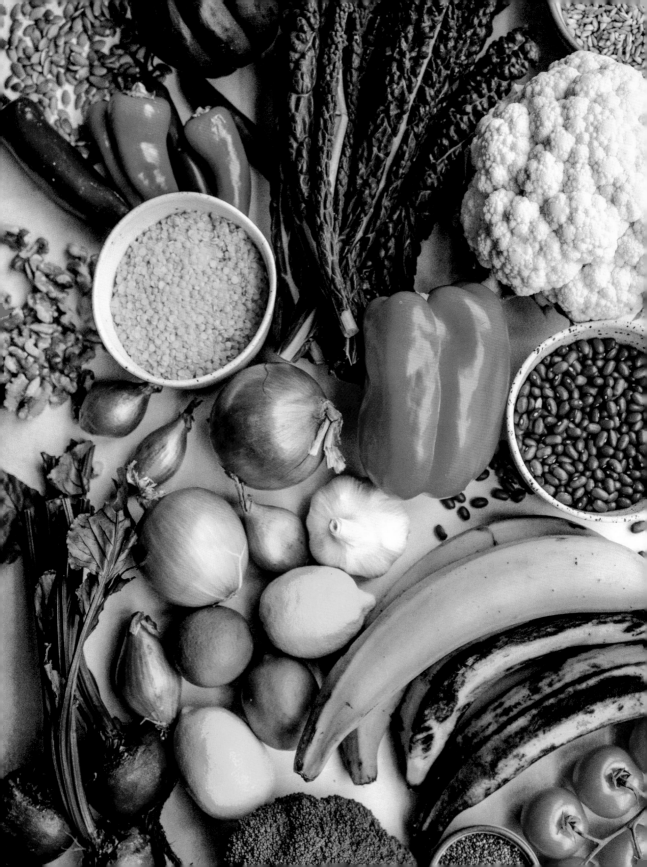

EASY PLANT-BASED PROTEIN SWAPS TO TRY:

- Replace dairy milk with soy milk for similar protein profiles.

- Try tofu in place of eggs to make tofu "egg" salad (see page 15).

- Use seitan (see page 137) to get that chew you might miss from meat.

- Use chickpeas in place of canned tuna in your "tuna" salad sandwiches (see page 75).

- Replace whey protein with a plant-based soy or pea-protein-based powder.

HEALTHY FATS

Don't be afraid of fats. Fats are an essential part of a healthy diet and are integral to many body functions including the absorption of vital nutrients and helping to cushion our vital organs.

When possible, aim to consume fats from whole food sources, as they have additional benefits including fiber, vitamins, and minerals. Whole fats include things like avocados, nuts (walnuts, almonds, pistachios, cashews, etc.), seeds (sunflower, pumpkin, chia, hemp, and flaxseeds), nut and seed butters, and olives. Be mindful of saturated fats, which can come from coconut and some processed foods that contain palm oil. Keeping saturated fat intake low may help lower the risk of developing heart disease.

DIETITIAN TIP

Aim to include at least one serving of an omega-3 rich fat. This includes ground flaxseeds, chia seeds, hemp hearts, or walnuts. You can prep your own Super Seed Mix (page 176). If you find this difficult to get in regularly, you may find benefit in using an algae-based supplement instead.

FILL IN THE GAPS

Eating a variety of nutrient-dense foods that include complex carbohydrates, fruits, vegetables, plant-based proteins, and healthy fats can satisfy our need for a lot of fiber, vitamins, and minerals. However, there still may be some nutrients that are easier to get using the following recommendations.

FORTIFIED FOODS

Including fortified foods in your diet will help to make hitting certain nutrient recommendations like calcium, vitamin B12, and vitamin D a lot easier.

Various fortified items, such as plant-based milks, some plant-based yogurts, cereals, and juices like orange juice, will vary when it comes to the nutrients they may provide. Just double-check the nutrition-facts label and ingredients to confirm whether these options are fortified and with how much. Typically, two to three servings of fortified foods can help with meeting some nutrient needs such as calcium.

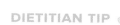

DIETITIAN TIP

You can meet your calcium needs by consuming at least three cups of any combination of calcium-fortified plant-based milks or juices, calcium-rich vegetables (kale, collards, bok choy, or turnip greens), or tofu that lists calcium sulfate in its ingredients.

IRON AND ZINC

By following the main recommendations, you will likely be consuming enough legumes, whole grains, nuts, and seeds that contain both minerals. However, it is important to note that these foods also contain compounds that may make absorbing iron and zinc a little more difficult. Accommodating for this is important.

DIETITIAN TIP

To enhance iron absorption, pair iron-rich foods with a good source of vitamin C like citrus fruits, mango, pineapple, strawberries, broccoli, Brussels sprouts, peppers, cabbage, and cauliflower. Pair zinc-rich foods like whole grains with sulfur-containing ingredients like onion and garlic to help increase zinc absorption by 50 percent!* Soaking and sprouting ingredients like beans and whole grains in water before cooking can also help remove inhibitors and enhance the absorption of these minerals.

---

* Janet R. Hunt, "Bioavailability of Iron, Zinc, and Other Trace Minerals from Vegetarian Diets," *American Journal of Clinical Nutrition* 78, suppl. 3 (September 2003): 633S–639S, https://doi.org/10.1093/ajcn/78.3.633S.

SHOULD YOU BE SUPPLEMENTING?

There is nothing wrong with supplementing when it's warranted. Sometimes it can be challenging to hit every single nutrient in a day with just food alone, whether you are vegan or not. Supplements, such as vitamin B12, vitamin D, or omega-3, are meant to supplement your diet and help fill in any gaps that can't be met by the foods you are eating. Just make sure you aren't taking more than you need and that you aren't wasting money on unnecessary supplements (this includes things like expensive greens powders and nutrients you likely get very easily with diet alone). There are a lot of people out there trying to sell something to you that you could probably live without. Always consult your own personal health care provider before making any changes to supplements.

Vitamin B12

Vitamin B12 is utilized by the body in the formation of red blood cells, DNA, and nervous system function. It is naturally found in foods of origin, which means that plant-based eaters *need* to obtain vitamin B12 from fortified foods and/or supplements.[*] This by no means makes a plant-based diet inferior. Some omnivores can become vitamin B12 deficient even with regular consumption of animal products, and as you age your body starts having a more difficult time absorbing this nutrient. Using supplements and fortified foods helps all these demographics meet their nutrient needs. As a plant-based eater, you can either use a daily B12 supplement of between 25 to 100 micrograms daily or 1,000 micrograms twice per week.

Vitamin D

Depending on where you live in the world and how often you are out in the sun, it might be difficult to synthesize enough vitamin D on your own. The normal recommendation is typically 600 IU per day, which can be achieved using fortified foods like plant-based milks and cereals or through supplementation. Regardless, always consult with your dietitian or doctor to see what is appropriate for you.

---

[*] "Vitamin B12: Fact Sheet for Health Professionals," National Institutes of Health, updated December 22, 2022, accessed October 8, 2023, https://ods.od.nih.gov/factsheets/VitaminB12-Health Professional/.

Iodine

This nutrient is often forgotten, but it is vital to help maintain a healthy thyroid. Half a teaspoon of iodized salt contains all the iodine you need in a day. You can alternatively supplement if you don't regularly use iodized salt at the table or when cooking.

KNOW YOUR NUTRIENTS

One way that you can get a better idea of the nutrients you are consuming in a day is to familiarize yourself with reading a food label. This is particularly helpful when it comes to navigating packaged foods and seeing how you want to fit them into your day-to-day eating habits.

While the numbers on a food label can seem overwhelming at first glance, there are just a few things you need to know to use it to your advantage.

SERVINGS: This just tells you how many servings are in the package. All the information on the nutrition label is based on a predetermined single serving. So, if you have a single serving of food, you will consume the nutrients listed on the package. If you happen to eat two servings, then you will be consuming double the nutrients listed on the label. Everyone's nutrient needs are different, so if you need more or less than contained in one suggested serving listed on a package, adjust accordingly.

DAILY VALUE: This is marked by the percentages listed on the label. The percentages are used as a tool to convey to consumers the level of a nutrient in a food in relation to an individual's requirement of that nutrient. While it's not a perfect system, this tool can still be used to tell you if a food product is low or high in a particular nutrient. These numbers can also help with comparing different products side by side, so you can choose the product that best suits your nutrient needs.

USE THE 5/20 RULE

The 5/20 rule is a general rule that can help you determine if a food is high or low in a nutrient.* This rule does not apply morality to food, but instead encourages nutrient

---

* "The Lows and Highs of Percent Daily Value on the Nutrition Facts Label," U.S. Food & Drug Administration, updated September 27, 2023, https://www.fda.gov/food/nutrition-facts-label/lows-and-highs-percent-daily-value-nutrition-facts-label/.

choices that can help reduce the risk for chronic disease. When looking at daily value (DV) percentages on a package, use this as a general rule:

5 PERCENT DV OR LESS indicates that a specific nutrient is low per serving. Nutrients that we generally want to keep low include saturated fat, sodium, and added sugars.

20 PERCENT DV OR MORE indicates that a specific nutrient is high per serving. Nutrients we generally want to be consuming more of in this category include fiber, vitamin D, calcium, iron, and potassium.

Reminder, nutrition labels are not designed to make you give up the foods you love. If anything, they can be a way to help you decide how you want to fit a specific food into your day-to-day life. For example, if you want to enjoy a food high in sodium, you may want to be mindful of your sodium intake with your remaining meals and use food labels to help. If you notice that you haven't consumed much fiber early in the day, you can pay closer attention and look for foods higher in fiber that can help you hit your daily requirement.

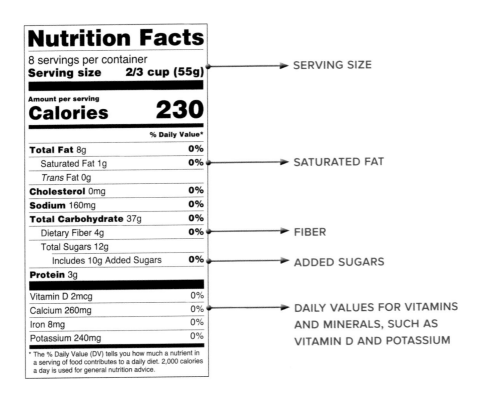

Equipment

You don't need fancy equipment to make good food. I say this as someone who is obsessed with kitchen gadgets. You truly only need a few basics to get by. I have found that everything else eventually just turns into clutter in your kitchen. So here are my most tried-and-true kitchen tools I use regularly.

HIGH-QUALITY KNIFE

The only knife you really need is a reliable chef's knife that you personally like. The size of the blade can vary slightly, but on average this knife is about 8 inches in length. Choose one with a sturdy handle you feel comfortable holding. And make sure you take care of it (hand wash, dry immediately, sharpen every one to two months depending on how often you use it) because this type of knife can last you a long time.

WHETSTONE

Over time with many uses, your knife will dull. A whetstone is a sharpening block that will help keep your knife sharp. Cutting with a dull knife might not sound so bad, but it most often leads to injury because a dull knife may slip as you try to cut through something. There is a productivity story about "sharpening your axe" that is used as a metaphor for how often we overwork ourselves, which leads to us not being our "sharpest" or most productive self. The story can also be taken quite literally in a culinary sense. Sharpening your knife will make chopping easier and faster, which will improve your kitchen experience significantly.

CUTTING BOARD

I like to keep two on hand in the kitchen. I use a small one for cutting up fruit or smaller foods that don't have a strong odor to them and a larger cutting board for everything else. Pro tip: keep a thin, damp paper towel or thin kitchen towel under your board to help prevent it from sliding as you are cutting.

HIGH-SPEED BLENDER

The type you get depends on the type of person you are. I am a fan of my Vitamix because it blends things ultrasmooth, including tougher-to-blend items like nuts. If you are only using your blender for things like simple sauces and easy-to-blend smoothies, you can do a lot with something cheaper like a Nutribullet.

FOOD PROCESSOR

A Cuisinart or Ninja food processor can be good options to include in your kitchen. If you don't have access to a food processor, then a handheld food chopper, an electric blender, an immersion blender, a grater, or simply a good knife and cutting board are affordable options that can be used alternatively depending on the recipe.

GOOD-QUALITY PANS

The type of pan I use depends on what I'm cooking. For the most part in this cookbook, I recommend a heavy-bottomed large skillet, a toxin-free medium nonstick pan, and a large saucepan. It also helps if you have lids for these pans. If you don't have a lid, you can get away with using a sheet pan to rest overtop your pot or pan as it cooks.

BAKING ESSENTIALS

Nothing too crazy here. You just need two nice large sheet pans, a muffin pan, and if you can fit it into your budget, a wire rack to cool any baked goods. For lining, I always use some form of parchment paper to make cleanup more bearable, especially on a busy weeknight.

MICROPLANE AND BOX GRATER

I use both at least once a day. I use the Microplane to zest citrus fruits and to finely grate garlic and ginger. The box grater is a wonderful option for shredding vegetables but can also be used to transform protein textures. I love to use mine to shred both tofu and tempeh, which gives you more surface area to flavor these proteins and to crisp them up in the oven.

CITRUS SQUEEZER

When I buy a tool, I want it to typically have more than one function, but I make an exception for my citrus squeezer. While you can often just squeeze citrus by hand, you likely won't get nearly as much juice out as you will when using this tool.

OVEN THERMOMETER

Sometimes ovens don't always get as hot as you think they do, which can play a big role in how a recipe turns out. I keep one in my oven at all times and use it to make sure the oven is indeed at the temperature I need it at.

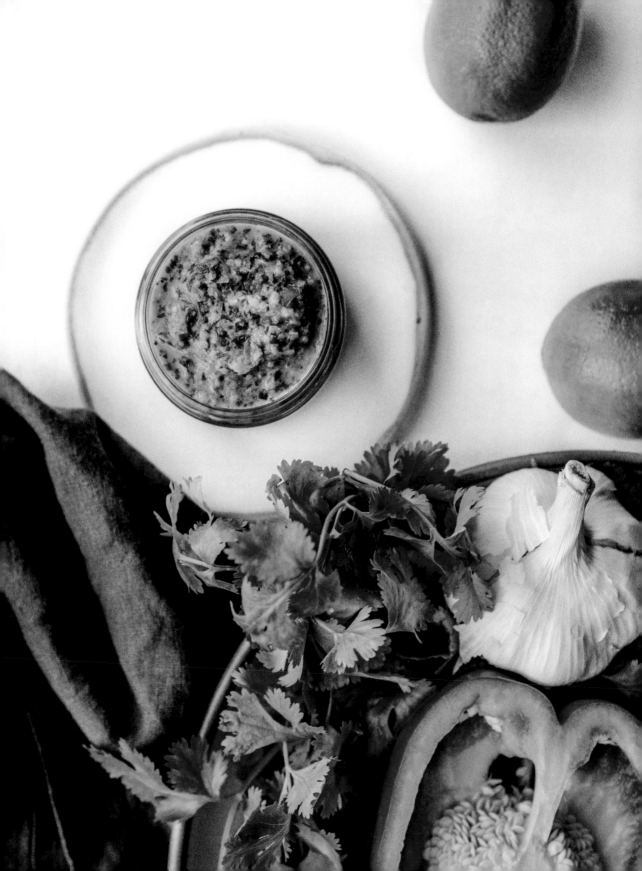

GARLIC PRESS

Depending on the type of person you are, this is a completely optional purchase. For me, I'm a garlic girl. If a recipe calls for one to three cloves, I will just use my Microplane to grate my garlic. Once it goes above that, I use a garlic press to mince all my garlic quickly.

STORAGE CONTAINERS

Make sure that the containers you use are practical and fit your needs. If you like to use them to microwave leftovers, make sure they are microwave safe. I also love jars for things like sauces, overnight oats, or mason jar–style grab-and-go salads. While you can buy expensive ones, I personally just save old glass peanut butter or jelly jars, clean them out, and repurpose them to use for storage. This also doubles as a way to give the food you store more personality, which in turn can make food prepping a little more fun and visually more exciting. It's the epitome of eating with your eyes.

KITCHEN UTENSILS

The ones I use the most are my silicone spatulas and whisk for stirring and mixing, a large spatula for flipping, a spoon to stir and ladle soups or stews, and tongs for more controlled tossing and item flipping.

KITCHEN SCALE

No fancy or expensive scale needed. I recommend getting an inexpensive one if you happen to love baking as much as I do. This will give you the most accurate measures when baking, which will lead to more consistent results. Plus, if you are measuring everything into one bowl, you have less to worry about when it comes to cleaning up.

Grocery Essentials

So you want to stock up on the plant-based essentials, but you aren't sure where to start. Luckily, not only is this list great to have if you are shopping for recipes in this cookbook, but it also provides some other general options to hopefully make your life more satisfying and full of flavor.

FRUITS

Apples

Apricots

Bananas

Blackberries

Blueberries

Cherries

Kiwis

Lemons

Limes

Mangoes

Medjool dates

Oranges

Peaches

Pears

Pineapples

Plums

Pomegranates

Raisins

Raspberries

Strawberries

Watermelon

VEGETABLES

Asparagus

Avocados

Beets

Bell peppers (any color)

Broccoli

Brussels sprouts

Cabbage

Carrots

Cauliflower

Corn

Cucumbers

Eggplant

Garlic

Ginger root

Green beans

Herbs, fresh (cilantro, parsley, dill, basil, etc.)

Kale

Leeks

Mushrooms

Onions (red, yellow, white, spring, etc.)

Plantains

Potatoes (Yukon gold, sweet potatoes, russet potatoes, etc.)

Radishes

Romaine lettuce

Shallots

Summer squash

Tomatoes

Winter squash (kabocha squash, butternut squash, acorn squash, etc.)

Zucchini

FREEZER-FRIENDLY ITEMS

Edamame

Frozen fruit (single fruit, mixed fruit, or berries)

Frozen vegetables (single vegetables or vegetable medley)

PANTRY STAPLES

Baking powder

Baking soda

Beans, canned or dried (black, kidney, white, pinto, chickpeas, etc.)

Chipotle peppers

Coconut milk, canned

Cornstarch

Farro

Flour (all-purpose, whole grain, or gluten-free)

Lentils, canned or dried

Millet

Noodles (soba, rice, or vermicelli)

Nutritional yeast

Oats (rolled, quick, or steel-cut)

Oils (olive, extra-virgin olive, avocado, sesame, etc.)

Pasta (whole grain, brown rice, or bean-based)

Potato starch

Quinoa

Rice (white, brown, or black)

Sugar (granulated, light brown, or coconut)

Tomatoes, canned or jarred

Tomato paste

Tortillas (corn or flour)

Vanilla extract

Vegan dark chocolate bars or chocolate chips

Vital wheat gluten

Whole grain or sourdough breads

NUTS & SEEDS

Almonds, natural almond butter

Cashews, natural cashew butter

Chia seeds

Flaxseeds (ground up for better nutrient absorption)

Hemp hearts

Peanuts, natural peanut butter

Pepitas

Pistachios

Sesame seeds

Sunflower seeds

Tahini

Walnuts

REFRIGERATED ITEMS

Miso paste (yellow or white)

Pickles

Plant-based cream cheese

Plant-based milk

Plant-based yogurt

Seitan

Tempeh

Tofu (silken, firm, extra-firm, super-firm)

Vegan kimchi

DRIED HERBS & SPICES

Adobo

Allspice

Basil

Bay leaves

Black pepper

Cardamom

Chili powder

Cinnamon

Coriander, (ground or seeds)

Cumin (ground or seeds)

Curry powder

Dill

Fennel seeds

Five-spice powder

Garam masala

Garlic powder

Dried herbs and spices (cont.)

Ginger (ground)	Parsley	Thyme
Italian seasoning	Red pepper flakes	Turmeric
Onion powder	Sazón	White pepper
Oregano	Smoked paprika	

CONDIMENTS

Agave syrup	Hummus	Soy sauce (tamari, low-sodium soy sauce, or coconut aminos)
BBQ sauce	Ketchup	
Buffalo sauce (dairy-free)	Maple syrup (pure)	Sriracha
Chili crisp oil		Sweet chili sauce
Garlic chili sauce	Mayonnaise (vegan)	Vegetable broth or vegetable bouillon
Gochujang	Mirin	
Hoisin sauce	Mustard	Vinegars (balsamic, apple cider, rice wine, red wine, etc.)
Hot sauce	Salsas	

NOTES ON SOME PLANT-BASED INGREDIENTS

SOY FOODS

Before we get into the types of soy food available, let's talk about it briefly. As good and nutritious as soy is, plus its long history of use by various populations around the world, soy has unfortunately gotten an unwarranted bad rap. This has led to it being one of the most well-researched foods. In short, a lot of the concern around soy is based on the fact that it contains isoflavones, which can be classified as phytoestrogens. While phytoestrogens can bind to estrogen receptors, phytoestrogens are not the same as estrogen and do not behave the same as estrogen in the body. At moderate amounts, soy is safe to consume with either neutral or potentially beneficial and protective effects to our health. For a very comprehensive look at the research available on soy and a breakdown into topics of concern regarding soy using extensive cited research, I highly recommend the soy article written by dietitian Jack Norris from the website Vegan Health.[*]

---

[*] Jack Norris, "Soy: Research," Vegan Health, updated March 2011, accessed October 8, 2023, https://veganhealth.org/soy/soy-part-2/.

Tofu

Tofu is the by-product of coagulated soy milk. The resulting curds are pressed together to form a tofu cake. How the tofu cake is pressed will determine the consistency of the tofu block you get. Here are the most common types of tofu you can find at your local market:

SILKEN TOFU: This form has the highest water content, making it soft and silky in texture, perfect for blending into smoothies or scooping or cubing into soups and stews.

FIRM AND EXTRA-FIRM TOFU: These blocks are pressed for a longer time, which creates a denser texture that holds its shape better. Firm is slightly softer than extra-firm, but both can be cut and tossed in marinades to add flavor and then sautéed or baked to make them chewier in texture.

SUPER-FIRM/HIGH-PROTEIN TOFU: This is the densest of the tofu varieties, which makes it extra meaty in texture. Typically, this tofu is stored in a vacuum-sealed package instead of the standard tub of water that firm and extra-firm tofu are often stored in. As a result, there is no need to drain or press water out of it, so it's ready to use straight out of the package. Compared to other types of tofu, it has the highest protein content per serving.

My go-to brands for tofu include Nasoya and House Foods.

Pressing and Draining Your Tofu

Straight out of the package, tofu can be saturated with a lot of water. For varieties such as firm or extra-firm that are used to sauté or bake, you may wish to press out additional water to help improve the taste and texture for its application. Here are three options you can use for pressing excess water out of your tofu:

1. PRESS WITH YOUR HANDS: Drain the extra-firm tofu right out of the package and give it a gentle squeeze while holding its shape to release some liquid, then pat dry with a clean towel. Your tofu will still have excess water in it, so it may dilute the flavor of sauces or seasonings used on it.

2. DIY TOFU PRESS: Press your tofu using things you already have at home. Remove the tofu from its container, wrap it in a clean kitchen towel, then sandwich the

wrapped tofu between two cutting boards or flat plates. Balance a heavy pot or book on top and allow to sit for fifteen to thirty minutes.

3. **COMMERCIAL TOFU PRESS**: If you like tofu and plan to use it regularly, you may wish to invest in a tofu press. Using a tofu press can help remove excess water from tofu without the mess or waste of extra paper towels. Simply place the tofu in the device and press as directed.

Tempeh

While in the same soy category as tofu, tempeh is very different in taste and consistency. Tempeh is a traditional Indonesian food made by fermenting whole, partially cooked soybeans with a tempeh starter. As it uses whole soybeans, the taste, texture, and nutrition profile of tempeh is different from tofu. It is high in protein and fiber, has a solid and firm texture, and typically has an earthy and nutty taste to it. For some, that flavor can be off-putting, especially if not cooked properly. Traditionally, tempeh is soaked in a brine or marinade and then fried or stir-fried. Just like with any food, when cooked and flavored well, tempeh is absolutely delicious.

PLANT-BASED DAIRY

Plant-Based Milks

You can find a lot of options in the plant-based milk aisle. My preference is to use soy milk since it is higher in protein than other plant-based milks, but feel free to use the unsweetened, plain version of the alternative milk you love instead.

Plant-Based Yogurt

There are a number of plant-based yogurts available on the market that will vary in consistency and taste based on the ingredients used. When choosing plant-based yogurts, use the one you like best. I generally use a plain, unsweetened cashew yogurt from Forager Project or a plain, unsweetened soy yogurt from Silk. You can also find good, thick coconut- and almond-based yogurts as well.

UMAMI-RICH INGREDIENTS

The following ingredients can be used to help add more savory, umami-rich flavors to your meal.

Nutritional Yeast

This is not the same as traditional yeast used for breads. Nutritional yeast is used in a lot of vegan recipes to add a lightly cheesy or richer umami flavor to a dish. It can also add more protein to meals and, when fortified, provides vitamin B12.

Miso Paste

Miso is a Japanese fermented soy paste. When added to dishes, it provides a rich umami flavor. In most of the recipes I share, I use a yellow or white miso paste. Both are interchangeable when it comes to this book. I would not swap yellow or white miso one to one for red miso paste as it has a very robust flavor and you would need to use less.

Tamari

Throughout this book you will see me reference tamari. This is a type of soy sauce that tends to be a little bit thicker and is often made with little or no wheat. For my gluten-free friends, since some tamari can be made with wheat, always double-check the label to ensure it is gluten-free before purchasing. In recipes, feel free to swap tamari for regular soy sauce, gluten-free soy sauce, or coconut aminos for a soy-free option.

Vegetable Broth

I like the seasoned vegetable Better than Bouillon base reconstituted in water or any of the Edward & Sons line of vegan vegetable, "chicken," or "beef" bouillon cubes prepared with the appropriate amount of water. You can alternatively use your favorite vegetable-broth cartons or make your own using vegetable scraps. Regardless of what you use, make sure it is good quality and adds a lot of flavor to your dishes.

BAKING INGREDIENTS

Aquafaba

Aquafaba is the liquid from a can of chickpeas or other beans. This may sound odd, but the starches in the liquid act similarly to how egg whites behave in baked goods. They act like a binder that provides lift and structure to baked goods. This is a great ingredient swap for baked goods that have a lighter crumb like cakes. Your cake won't taste like chickpeas, promise!

Whole Wheat Pastry Flour

If you plan to swap out all-purpose flour in a recipe, be mindful that it will impact the result of your recipe. All-purpose flour is light and also contains gluten, which gives you a consistent result when baking. If you are not gluten-free and looking for a way to increase fiber, a good swap for some recipes might be to use whole wheat pastry flour. This type of flour is ground and sifted more, yielding a lighter consistency that performs much better in baking compared to regular whole wheat flour.

Meal Prep Smarter, Not Harder

As a dietitian, I am not here to tell you exactly what you need to eat every day. What I am here to do is to help make those decisions easier. Meal planning in general can support you in the following ways:

- Help you save money

- Keep your meals nutritious and balanced

- Can help you save time

- Cause less stress because you already know "what's for dinner"

- Provide meals to look forward to

CONSIDER THESE THINGS BEFORE YOU START PLANNING

MANAGE YOUR DECISION FATIGUE

We are presented with hundreds of choices in a given day, and then we have to decide what to eat for dinner. That's brutal. I like to keep a list of my favorite foods that I don't get tired of, and on days where I can't be bothered to think, I refer to it and use it to help guide me in making a decision. This list typically includes just three breakfast ideas, three lunch ideas, and three dinner ideas. I keep the list small to avoid getting overwhelmed and then will rotate recipes as needed every few weeks.

YOU DON'T HAVE TO PREP FULL MEALS

I mean you technically can prep full meals, but I find that if you are prepping one recipe to last over four to five days, you may very likely get bored of it by day two. By day eight when you finally remember it's in the back of the fridge, it might have already turned into a science experiment. Instead, prep with purpose and with the knowledge that your plans may pivot. What this means is, think of what you want to eat for the week, and prep the most time-consuming elements in advance. For example, don't wait until the day of to press your tofu. That can eat up thirty minutes of your time on a busy weeknight. When planning meals, consider taking a moment during the week to press that tofu. You can also do the following:

PREP ALL YOUR LEGUMES. This can include cooking a large batch of beans from scratch (stove or pressure cooker) or draining and drying off canned beans and storing in the fridge so it saves you a step when you're ready to cook.

COOK YOUR GRAINS. Cook them in advance and store in the fridge. You can also double-batch and freeze some for later. A rice cooker can be a great investment if you also want less guesswork with cooking your grains perfectly.

GET YOUR SAUCES IN ORDER. I like to make one to two sauces at the start of the week. Once prepped, they can last a few days in the fridge and can make a relatively boring meal more flavorful.

MAXIMIZE YOUR CUTTING BOARD TIME. If you are already using your cutting board, take a minute to prep and cut some extra vegetables for the next day.

Just these little things alone can help you save a significant amount of time in the kitchen during the workweek. It's like having half your recipe completed before you start. On top of that, it allows you the opportunity to enjoy fresher food. No one likes day three of one meal, let alone day four.

IT'S OKAY TO HAVE HELP

In an ideal world I would love for everyone to have access to plenty of time and to make everything from scratch, but that's not realistic. Keep these ideas in mind to help save time in the kitchen:

- Feel free to use prechopped veggies.

- Use a veggie chopper if you hate chopping.

- Frozen and canned items can be a huge time-saver.

- Microwavable precooked shelf-stable grains and noodles mean you don't have to dirty another pot.

- Get others involved in the kitchen where it makes sense—have friends or family help with chopping, prewashing, and measuring things out.

FOOD STORAGE TIPS

You've spent all this time making this food, so let's make sure it is stored properly—we want to make the most of the food you have, as well as keep you safe. Store properly cooled foods in airtight containers in the fridge or freezer depending on a recipe's instructions. Recommended storage date ranges are based on guidelines from FoodSafety.gov. These standards are put in place to help prevent the development of foodborne illness. When following storage recommendations, keep in mind that food meant to be stored in the fridge should not sit out longer than two hours at room temperature. Any longer at room temperature and you start increasing the risk for harmful bacteria to grow in your food. These guidelines might seem "extra," and maybe you've been lucky enough not to have dealt with getting sick from something like this, but the risk exists—and the consequences are not worth it.

CHAPTER 1

This is your FIRST OPPORTUNITY of the day to provide your body with NOURISHMENT. Whether it's savory or sweet, here are some ideas to help you POWER UP your mornings.

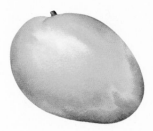

Breaking the Fast

Smoothies give you an opportunity to load up on a lot of nourishing ingredients. Prep the ingredients in advance to make smoothie pouches that you can store in the freezer. When you are ready to have a smoothie, all you have to do is dump the bag in the blender cup, add any extras, and blend it up to creamy perfection. Here are four of my absolute favorite smoothie combos that also help you sneak in some veggies.

Ready, Set, Smoothies

Blueberry Muffin Smoothie

SERVES 1 · PREP TIME: 10 MINUTES

For as simple as this smoothie is, when I first took a sip of it, I felt like I was sitting outside of a bakery munching on a blueberry muffin. A bold thing to say about a humble smoothie, but I mean it! It tastes that good and still manages to sneak in zucchini without you knowing it's there. The bonus of adding the frozen zucchini is that it will make the smoothie creamier and also load it up with additional antioxidants.

FOR THE FREEZER BAG

1 cup frozen blueberries

½ ripe banana, sliced

½ small zucchini roughly chopped (about ½ cup)

¼ cup gluten-free rolled oats

Zest of ½ lemon

FOR BLENDING

1 soft Medjool date, pit removed

1 tablespoon natural almond butter

½ teaspoon ground cinnamon

1 cup unsweetened soy milk

Pinch of kosher salt

PREPARE THE FREEZER BAG

To a freezer bag, add the blueberries, banana, zucchini, rolled oats, and lemon zest. Place the bag in the freezer for at least 8 hours or overnight.

BLEND THE SMOOTHIE

When ready to prepare the smoothie, add the contents of the freezer bag to a high-speed blender cup along with the date, almond butter, cinnamon, soy milk, and salt. Blend on high until completely smooth, then serve.

 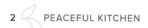

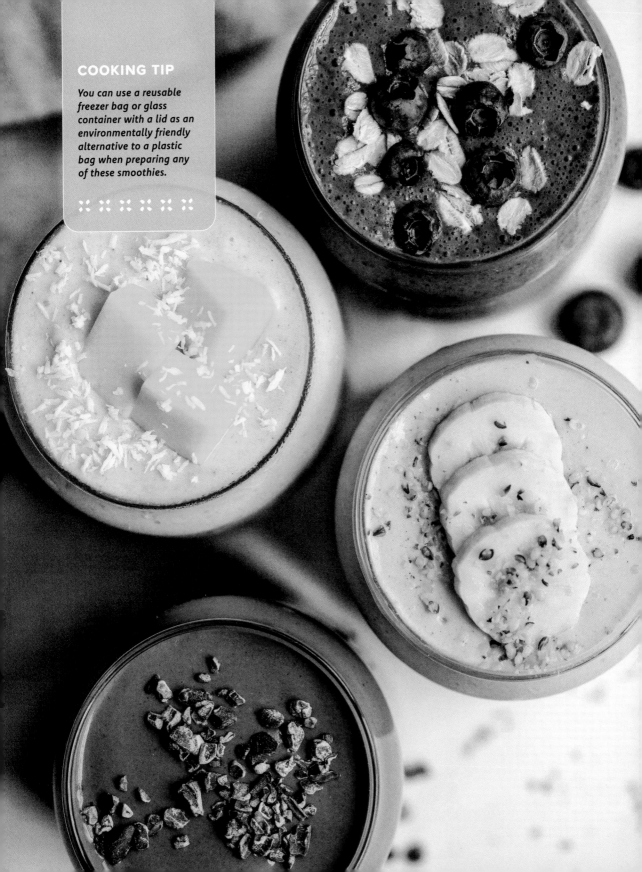

COOKING TIP

You can use a reusable freezer bag or glass container with a lid as an environmentally friendly alternative to a plastic bag when preparing any of these smoothies.

Zesty Mango Lime Smoothie

SERVES 1 • PREP TIME: 10 MINUTES

Mango and Tajín belong together. It's a flavor pairing I've grown up enjoying, made popular by Mexican fruit vendors. Their fruit cups were the thing I looked forward to the most once the weather got warmer. One of my favorite flavors to order was mango sprinkled with some Tajín, sometimes some chamoy, a sauce made from dried fruit and chili peppers. It's the perfect combination of sweet, tangy citrus, and salty, so turning this into a smoothie was a must.

Over the years, I have tweaked this recipe to add more protein and to give an extra boost of antioxidants by including some turmeric, which contains the antioxidant curcumin. Historically this spice is used in Ayurvedic practices, and some studies show benefit in reducing inflammation caused by a range of different conditions. If you want that benefit, it is best to pair turmeric with a little black pepper, which helps improve absorption of curcumin by 2,000 percent.*

FOR THE FREEZER BAG

1 cup frozen mango chunks

½ ripe banana, sliced

½ cup zucchini, chopped

3 tablespoons hemp hearts

1 tablespoon coconut flakes

½ teaspoon lime zest

FOR BLENDING

1 soft Medjool date, pit removed

1 cup unsweetened soy milk

¼ teaspoon Tajín or chili-lime seasoning, plus more for serving

¼ teaspoon ground turmeric

Pinch of freshly ground black pepper

PREPARE THE FREEZER BAG

To a freezer bag, add the mango, banana, zucchini, hemp hearts, coconut flakes, and lime zest. Place in the freezer for at least 8 hours or overnight.

BLEND THE SMOOTHIE

When ready to prepare the smoothie, add the contents of the freezer bag to a blender cup along with the date, soy milk, Tajín, turmeric, and black pepper. Blend until completely smooth, then serve with an extra dusting of Tajín on top.

---

* G. Shoba, D. Joy, T. Joseph, M. Majeed, R. Rajendran, and P. S. Srinivas, "Influence of Piperine on the Pharmacokinetics of Curcumin in Animals and Human Volunteers," *Planta Medica* 64, no. 4 (1998): 353–56, https://doi.org/10.1055/s-2006–957450.

Salted Tahini Date Smoothie

SERVES 1 • PREP TIME: 10 MINUTES

One of my all-time favorite shakes I ever had was at a small place called Goldie in Philadelphia. The base of the shake uses tahini, and when blended you get the most incredible creamy, sweet blend of deliciousness. I swear it changes lives and makes you want to use a good-quality tahini in everything. And maybe that's a good thing because the minerals found in tahini help support bone health. Now, between that, the banana, and the dates, you won't notice the cauliflower added. Yes, I snuck that in to help you get some veggies at the start of your day. I know it sounds weird, but it works, just trust me!

FOR THE FREEZER BAG

1 ripe banana, sliced

½ cup frozen cauliflower

¼ cup gluten-free rolled oats

1 tablespoon coconut flakes

1 tablespoon hemp hearts

FOR BLENDING

2 soft Medjool dates, pits removed

2 tablespoons good-quality tahini (see page 59)

½ teaspoon ground cinnamon

Pinch of ground cardamom

Pinch of kosher salt

1 cup unsweetened soy milk

PREPARE THE FREEZER BAG

To a freezer bag, add the banana, cauliflower, rolled oats, coconut flakes, and hemp hearts. Place in the freezer for at least 8 hours or overnight.

BLEND THE SMOOTHIE

When ready to blend the smoothie, add the contents of the freezer bag to a blender cup along with the dates, tahini, cinnamon, cardamom, salt, and soy milk. Blend on high until completely smooth. Serve immediately.

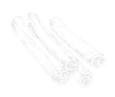

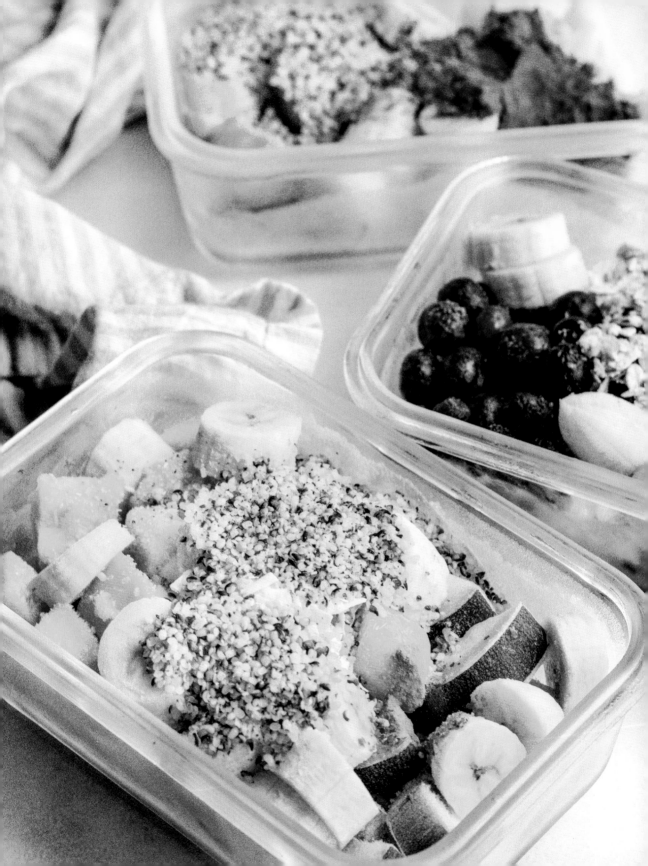

Creamy Chocolate Cardamom Smoothie

SERVES 1 • PREP TIME: 10 MINUTES

Okay, if the smoothie ain't thick, I don't want it. That is my smoothie rule. This one comes out extra creamy thanks to the addition of some heart-healthy avocado. Once you blend it all together with some cocoa powder, dates, and a banana, it feels more like an ultrarich chocolate shake. And I'm always happy to enjoy that for breakfast.

FOR THE FREEZER BAG

1 ripe banana, sliced

½ cup frozen cauliflower

¼ avocado, cubed

3 tablespoons hemp hearts

FOR BLENDING

2 soft Medjool dates, pits removed

2 tablespoons cocoa powder

¼ teaspoon ground cardamom

Pinch of kosher salt

1¼ cups unsweetened soy milk

PREPARE THE FREEZER BAG

To a freezer bag, add the banana, cauliflower, avocado, and hemp hearts. Place in the freezer for at least 8 hours or overnight.

BLEND THE SMOOTHIE

When ready to blend the smoothie, add the contents of the freezer bag to a blender cup with the dates, cocoa powder, cardamom, salt, and soy milk. Blend on high until completely smooth, then enjoy!

If you're getting bored with your typical oats, let's spice things up with four different tasty flavors. You can prep all four ahead of time and have different flavors to choose from over the course of the week. Good for up to four days in the fridge.

Overnight Oats Four Ways

Lemon Poppy Seed Overnight Oats

SERVES 1 • PREP TIME: 10 MINUTES

This easy-to-put-together recipe is for those mornings you want something fresh, zingy, and filling. The lemon really comes through and makes the oats taste like lemon poppy seed muffin batter. Let me recommend not eating muffin batter and instead giving these oats a try!

½ cup gluten-free rolled oats

1 tablespoon chia seeds

1 teaspoon poppy seeds

Pinch of kosher salt

¾ cup unsweetened soy milk

2 tablespoons plain unsweetened, plant-based yogurt

1 tablespoon maple syrup

Zest and juice of ½ lemon, plus more for serving

Fresh blueberries or Lemon Blueberry Chia Jam (page 224), for serving (optional)

To an airtight container, add the rolled oats, chia seeds, poppy seeds, and salt, then stir to combine.

To the same container, add the soy milk, yogurt, maple syrup, and lemon zest and juice, and stir well to combine. Allow the mixture to sit for 10 minutes, then stir well to prevent the chia seeds from clumping.

Seal the container and place in the fridge for at least 1 hour or overnight.

When ready to serve, stir well, then top with blueberries or jam and additional lemon zest, if desired. The oats can be stored in the fridge for up to 4 days.

COOKING TIP

Transform the Lemon Poppy Seed Overnight Oats into a Key lime pie version using Key limes. Fresh, vibrant, and delicious.

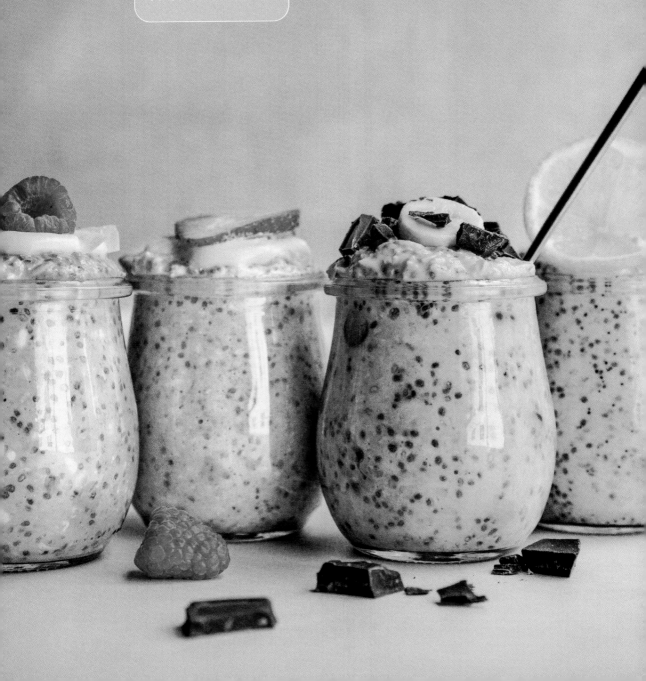

Strawberry Shortcake Overnight Oats

SERVES 1 • PREP TIME: 10 MINUTES

If you truly want to transform your experience with overnight oats, you need to blend the fruit into the milk before adding it to the oats. It helps give each bite of your oats that delicious fruity flavor that you are looking for. So when I say strawberry oats, I mean that I want each bite to taste like strawberries. And these oats definitely won't disappoint.

⅓ cup fresh or frozen strawberries

1 tablespoon strawberry jam

½ cup unsweetened soy milk

2 tablespoons plain unsweetened plant-based yogurt

1 soft Medjool date, pit removed

1 tablespoon chia seeds

1 tablespoon hemp hearts

Pinch of kosher salt

½ cup gluten-free rolled oats

2 strawberries, diced

1 tablespoon strawberry jam

Dollop of plant-based coconut whipped cream or plain unsweetened, plant-based yogurt (optional)

To a blender cup, add the strawberries, jam, soy milk, yogurt, date, chia seeds, hemp hearts, and salt. Blend the mixture on high until creamy and smooth.

In an airtight container, place the rolled oats and pour the strawberry mixture over top, then stir to fully combine.

For the topping, place the strawberries in a small bowl and mash with a fork. Stir in the jam, then pour the mixture over the oats.

Feel free to top with a dollop of your favorite plant-based coconut whipped cream, if desired, and enjoy. The oats can be stored in the fridge for up to 4 days.

Chocolate Chip Cookie Dough Oats

SERVES 1 • PREP TIME: 10 MINUTES

Cookies for breakfast? Kind of! Normally, I'm good with regular oats in the morning. But there are those days where I do crave something sweet when I wake up. For those mornings, this is my go-to. The almond butter really helps give these oats that cookie-dough vibe. And even if you wouldn't want something like this for breakfast, it's good enough as a sweet snack later in the day.

½ cup gluten-free rolled oats

1 tablespoon chia seeds

Pinch of kosher salt

¾ cup unsweetened soy milk

2 tablespoons plain unsweetened, plant-based yogurt

1 tablespoon natural almond butter or cashew butter, plus more for serving

1 tablespoon maple syrup

½ teaspoon vanilla extract

1 tablespoon chocolate chips, plus more for serving

Banana (optional)

To an airtight container, add the oats, chia seeds, and salt, then stir to combine.

Pour in the soy milk, yogurt, almond butter, maple syrup, vanilla, and chocolate chips, then stir again, making sure that the chia seeds don't clump. Allow the mixture to sit for 5 minutes, stir once more, then store in the fridge for up to 4 days.

Enjoy as is or top with extra chocolate chips, banana, and nut butter.

Matcha Cheesecake Overnight Oats

SERVES 1 • PREP TIME: 10 MINUTES

If you know me, you know I don't start the day without a matcha in some form. If you aren't familiar with it, matcha is derived from the grinding of green tea leaves. This makes it different than regular green tea in the sense that you are consuming the whole leaf. I love that it provides a stable level of energy, increased focus and attention, [*] *and lots of protective antioxidants as well. Infusing it into oats was a no-brainer, and combining those warm, earthy flavors of matcha into a cheesecake-flavored version was a must—the perfect meal to perk you up first thing in the morning.*

½ cup gluten-free rolled oats

1 tablespoon chia seeds

Pinch of kosher salt

1 teaspoon ceremonial-grade matcha (see Nutrition Tip)

2 tablespoons plant-based cream cheese, room temperature

1 tablespoon maple syrup

Zest of ½ lemon

2 teaspoons lemon juice

¾ cup unsweetened soy milk

Fresh fruit, for serving

To an airtight container, add the oats, chia seeds, and salt. Sift in the matcha using a small mesh sieve to ensure there are no clumps, then stir all the dry ingredients together.

In a large measuring cup or separate bowl, whisk together the cream cheese, maple syrup, lemon zest and juice, and soy milk until smooth.

Pour the mixture over the oats and whisk together to evenly mix. Allow the oats to sit for 10 minutes, then stir well again to make sure the chia seeds are not clumped together.

Seal the container and place in the fridge for at least 1 hour or overnight. When ready to serve, stir well, then top with fresh fruit and enjoy. The oats can be stored in the fridge for up to 4 days.

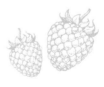

---

*   T. Giesbrecht, J. A. Rycroft, M. J. Rowson, and E. A. De Bruin, "The Combination of L-theanine and Caffeine Improves Cognitive Performance and Increases Subjective Alertness," *Nutritional Neuroscience* 13, no. 6 (2010): 283–90, https://doi.org/10.1179/147683010X12611460764840.

 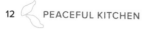

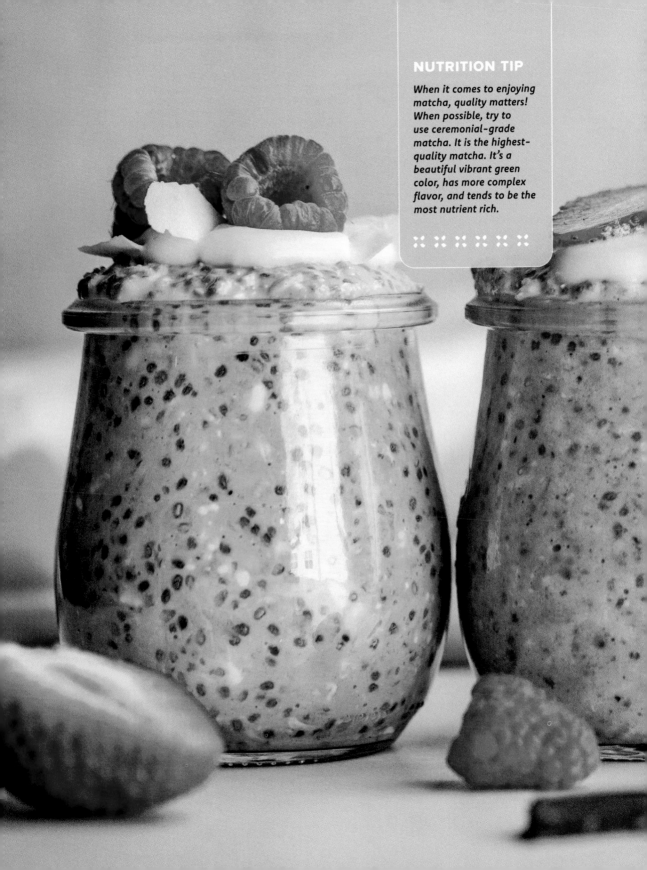

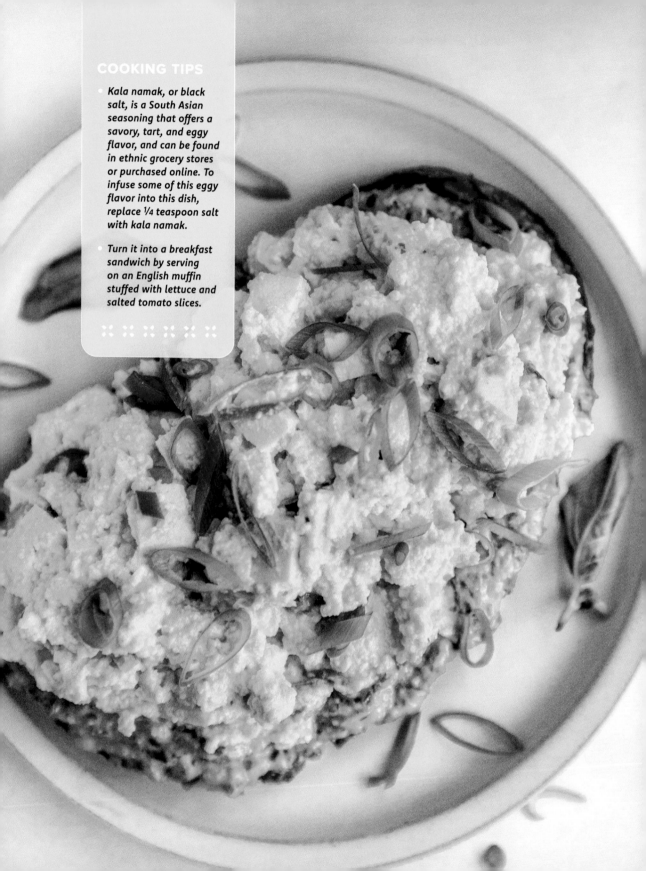

COOKING TIPS

• *Kala namak, or black salt, is a South Asian seasoning that offers a savory, tart, and eggy flavor, and can be found in ethnic grocery stores or purchased online. To infuse some of this eggy flavor into this dish, replace ¼ teaspoon salt with kala namak.*

• *Turn it into a breakfast sandwich by serving on an English muffin stuffed with lettuce and salted tomato slices.*

I will always be a big fan of the tofu scramble. When done right, it can be the perfect balance of fluffy, savory goodness to take my time with on the weekend. And that's kind of the problem with them—they require time that I generally don't have during the workweek. To fix this problem, I started meal prepping this tofu "egg" salad instead. It still gives me that eggy fix, but it's more convenient since I can prep it ahead of time. That means all I have to do in the morning is toast some bread and layer this on. Satisfying and packed with protein, this toast will make you excited to get up in the morning.

Pesto "Egg" Salad Breakfast Toast

SERVES 4 • PREP TIME: 10 MINUTES • COOKING TIME: 3 MINUTES

FOR THE "EGG" SALAD

1 16-ounce block firm tofu, drained and pressed (see page xxxix)

1/3 cup vegan mayonnaise

1 tablespoon lemon juice

2 teaspoons Dijon mustard

1 tablespoon nutritional yeast

1/4 teaspoon ground turmeric

1/2 teaspoon kosher salt

Freshly ground black pepper to taste

2 scallions, thinly sliced, plus more for serving

FOR SERVING

Sourdough, whole grain, or gluten-free bread, sliced

Charred Scallion Pesto (page 212)

PREPARE THE "EGG" SALAD

Cut the block of tofu in half. Finely dice one half of the tofu into 1/4-inch pieces and set aside. Place the remaining half of the tofu in a medium mixing bowl and mash it well using a fork until the tofu is uniformly crumbled.

To the bowl, add the mayonnaise, lemon juice, mustard, nutritional yeast, turmeric, salt, black pepper, and 1 tablespoon water. Use a spatula to mix the ingredients together evenly.

Add the cubed tofu and scallions and carefully fold them into the mixture, then adjust salt and pepper to taste. This mixture can be stored in an airtight container in the fridge for up to 5 days.

TO SERVE

Toast a slice of bread, then spread with 1 to 2 tablespoons of pesto. Layer on the tofu "egg" salad and garnish with extra scallions as desired before serving.

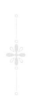

If you struggle getting enough plant-based protein at breakfast, then I want you to become a bigger fan of tempeh. You can get up to 18 grams of protein per serving, plus lots of fiber and iron. One of my favorite ways to enjoy tempeh in the morning is to turn it into a high-protein hash infused with some of the smoky sweet flavors that you would typically find in breakfast sausage. The best way to infuse those flavors is to mince the tempeh into very small pieces—I like to use a box grater to help with this—then it can be pan-fried and coated in a delicious range of sauces and spices. Make this ahead of time for the week and you have an easy high-protein option you can enjoy first thing in the morning.

Smoky Maple Tempeh Hash

SERVES 3 • PREP TIME: 15 MINUTES • COOKING TIME: 15 MINUTES

1 8-ounce block of tempeh

1 tablespoon tamari (see page xli)

1 tablespoon maple syrup

1 tablespoon apple cider vinegar

1 teaspoon smoked paprika

½ teaspoon ground coriander

½ teaspoon fennel seeds

½ teaspoon dried basil

¼ teaspoon ground cumin

1½ tablespoons avocado oil

Kosher salt to taste

1 shallot, minced

2 garlic cloves, minced

1 cup frozen corn, thawed

Use a box grater over a cutting board to grate the tempeh using the largest holes. If any large pieces remain, mince well with a knife. In a small bowl, combine the tamari, maple syrup, vinegar, paprika, coriander, fennel seeds, basil, and cumin, then whisk together and set aside.

To a large skillet, add 1 tablespoon of the oil, and place it over medium heat. Once the oil is hot, add the tempeh along with a pinch of salt and toss to coat. Spread the tempeh out on the pan into a single layer, then allow the tempeh to cook undisturbed for 2 minutes. Give the tempeh a toss and continue to cook, stirring occasionally, for 4 to 5 minutes until it has become golden in color, then transfer to a bowl.

Add the remaining ½ tablespoon of the oil to the pan to warm through, then add the shallot with a pinch of salt. Sauté the shallot for 1 to 2 minutes until softened, then add the garlic and sauté until fragrant, about 1 minute.

Stir in the thawed corn, then cook for 1 to 2 minutes until warmed through.

Add the cooked tempeh back to the skillet, then pour in the tamari mixture from earlier. Toss to combine and continue sautéing until the tempeh has absorbed all the liquid and is evenly mixed.

Remove from heat and serve immediately or store in an airtight container in the fridge for up to 5 days.

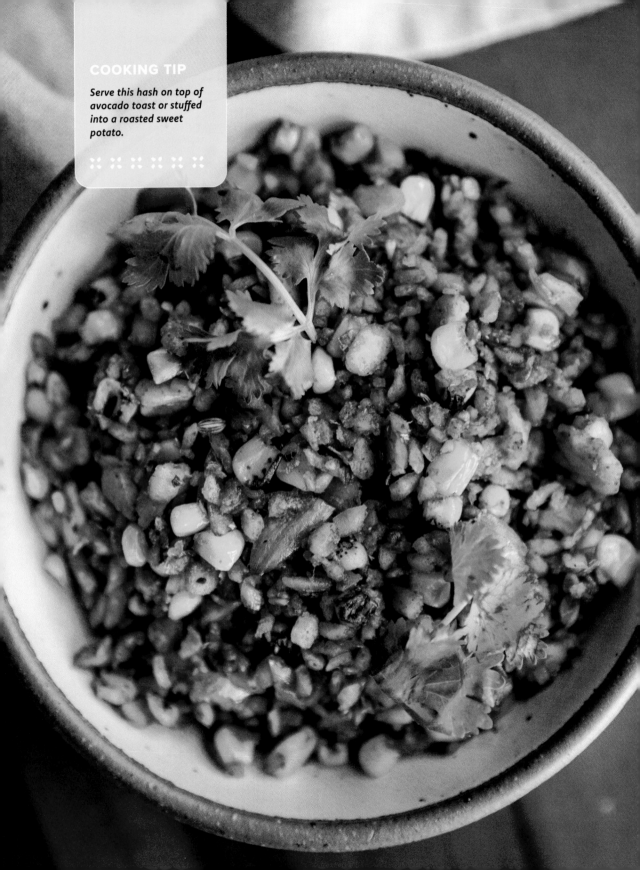

COOKING TIP

Serve this hash on top of avocado toast or stuffed into a roasted sweet potato.

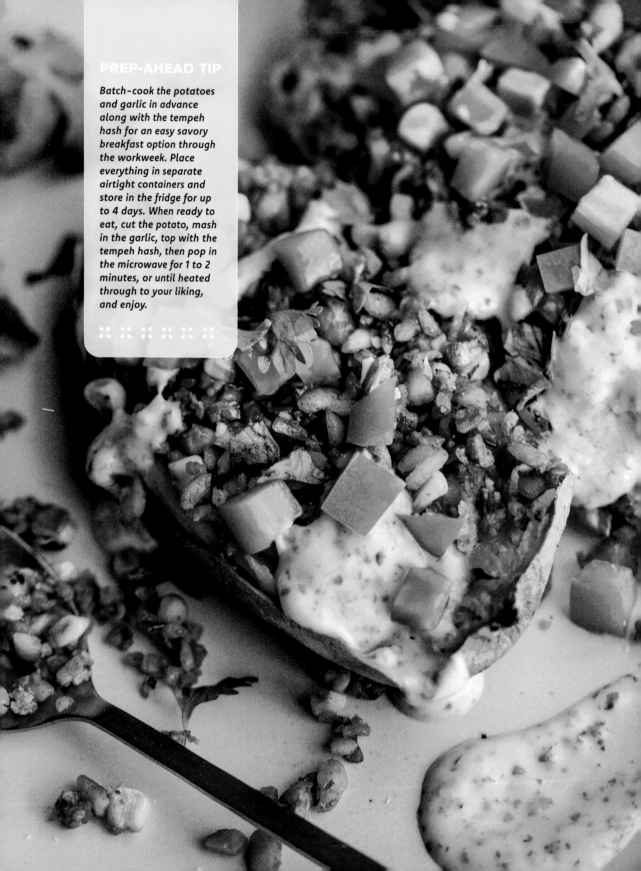

PREP-AHEAD TIP

Batch-cook the potatoes and garlic in advance along with the tempeh hash for an easy savory breakfast option through the workweek. Place everything in separate airtight containers and store in the fridge for up to 4 days. When ready to eat, cut the potato, mash in the garlic, top with the tempeh hash, then pop in the microwave for 1 to 2 minutes, or until heated through to your liking, and enjoy.

I'm not over avocado toast, but I, too, love variety. After making the Smoky Maple Tempeh Hash (page 16), I felt like it belonged stuffed in a perfectly roasted potato and drizzled with sauce and veggies. So here we are, roasting sweet potatoes, and you can totally make this for a fun Sunday brunch or batch-prep this for an easy-to-put together breakfast or dinner during the workweek. I leave that decision up to you.

Sweet Potato Boats

SERVES 3 • PREP TIME: 10 MINUTES • COOKING TIME: 55 MINUTES

3 medium sweet potatoes

1 small garlic head

1 teaspoon avocado oil

Kosher salt to taste

1 batch Smoky Maple Tempeh Hash (page 16)

Optional Topping Ideas: sliced avocado, diced plum tomatoes, Everything Sauce (page 220), or Avocado Pico de Gallo (page 206)

Preheat the oven to 425°F. Line a baking sheet with parchment paper.

Wash and scrub the outside of each sweet potato really well, then carefully poke a few holes over the surface with a fork and place them on the prepared tray.

Cut the top off of the garlic head and place on a sheet of foil. Drizzle the oil over the exposed cloves, then sprinkle with a pinch of salt. Wrap the garlic in the foil and place on the tray with the potatoes.

Place the baking sheet in the oven. Roast for 40 minutes, then remove the garlic and set aside. Return the tray to the bottom rack of the oven and roast for an additional 10 to 15 minutes or until the potatoes have cooked through.

Cut the sweet potatoes in half and squeeze 2 to 3 roasted garlic cloves on each side with a pinch of salt. Using a fork, lightly mash the garlic into the potatoes, add a third of the tempeh hash, then top as desired. Try this with a few slices of avocado, chopped tomatoes, a drizzle of Everything Sauce, or some Avocado Pico de Gallo, if desired.

Flavor and antioxidants: It's a true win when you can have both. Antioxidants help to neutralize free radicals that can cause oxidation in the body. We don't want oxidation because that can be harmful to our bodies and even lead to chronic disease. The more often you can sneak in some additional antioxidants, the better. So why not at breakfast? With this one you're getting a large variety of powerful antioxidants from both the raspberries and matcha. A truly powerful combo to start your day—and the rest of your life—off on the right foot.

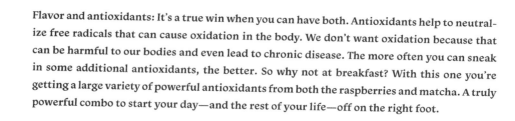

Raspberry Matcha Chia Pudding

SERVES 3 • PREP TIME: 20 MINUTES

FOR THE PUDDING

2 teaspoons ceremonial-grade matcha (see page 13)

½ cup hot water, no more than 180°F

¾ cup unsweetened soy milk

¼ cup plain unsweetened plant-based yogurt

2 tablespoons maple syrup

½ teaspoon vanilla extract

¼ teaspoon ground cardamom

¼ teaspoon kosher salt

⅓ cup chia seeds

FOR THE RASPBERRY LAYER

1 cup fresh or frozen raspberries, thawed

½ cup plain unsweetened plant-based yogurt

1 tablespoon chia seeds

1 tablespoon maple syrup (optional)

1 teaspoon lemon zest (optional)

FOR SERVING

Fresh fruit (optional)

PREPARE THE PUDDING

Using a small mesh sieve, sift your matcha into a medium mixing bowl, then pour in the hot water. Use a matcha whisk to whisk the matcha back and forth in a W-shape motion for about 1 minute. The matcha should be fully suspended in the water with froth on top.

To a medium mixing bowl, add the soy milk, yogurt, maple syrup, vanilla, cardamom, salt, and the matcha mixture, then whisk together until smooth.

Add the chia seeds, then whisk the mixture together to combine and set aside for at least 10 minutes.

PREPARE THE RASPBERRY LAYER

Add the thawed raspberries to a small mixing bowl and mash them completely using a fork. Once fully mashed, add the yogurt and chia seeds, as well as the maple syrup and lemon zest, if desired. Stir together to combine and set aside for at least 10 minutes.

After 10 minutes pass, stir both bowls separately to make sure the chia seeds have not clumped together. Transfer the matcha chia pudding and raspberry yogurt mixture into separate airtight containers and place in the fridge for at least 1 hour or overnight.

TO SERVE

Portion out a third of the chia pudding mixture and top with a third of the raspberry yogurt mixture. Top with extra fresh fruit if desired, then enjoy.

 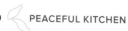

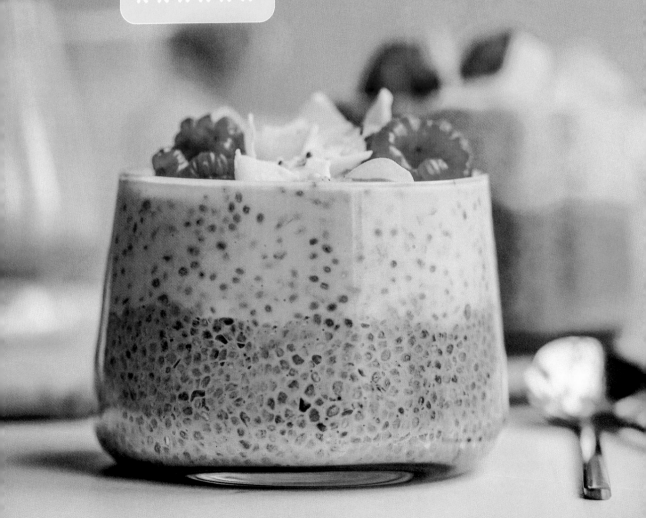

COOKING TIP

A matcha whisk is a traditional Japanese bamboo whisk used to evenly suspend matcha powder in water and aerate it. If you do not have a matcha whisk, you can use a handheld electric milk frother or blender to blend the matcha together with all the liquid ingredients to get a similar effect.

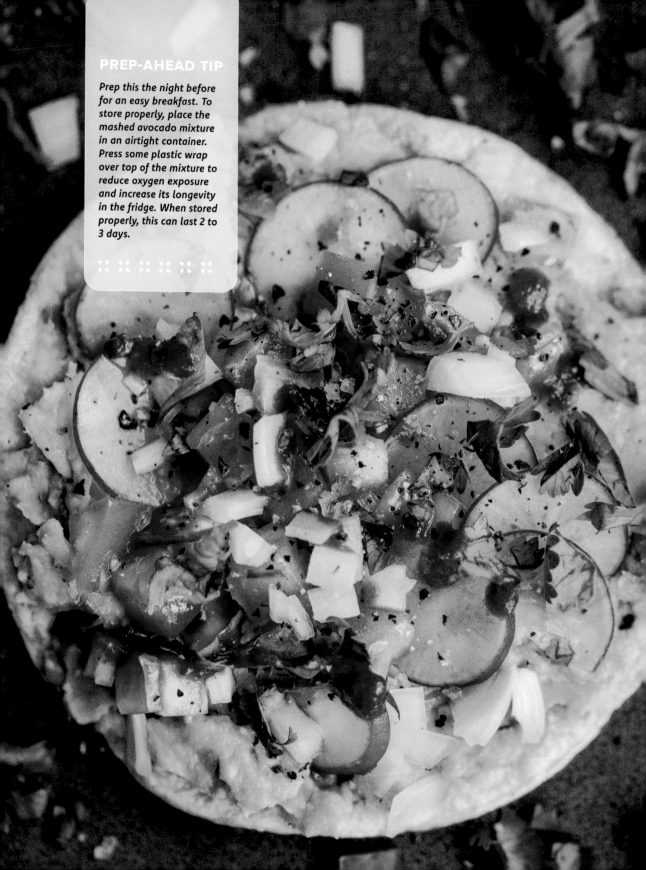

My heart will always belong to tostadas. So when I want to change up my morning bowl of oats, I will most often go to these breakfast tostadas. You can make the filling the night before—that way, you can just toast up some tortillas and spread with your avocado spread. And don't worry, it's packed with protein and fiber so that you will feel fueled up and energized.

Breakfast Tostadas

SERVES 3 • PREP TIME: 15 MINUTES • COOKING TIME: 6 MINUTES

6 corn tortillas

2 teaspoons avocado oil

Kosher salt to taste

1 15-ounce can cannellini beans, drained and rinsed

1 medium avocado

2 marinated artichoke hearts, minced

1 clove garlic, grated

Zest and juice of 1 lime

Freshly ground black pepper to taste

Pinch of everything seasoning blend

1 plum tomato, diced

2 tablespoons white onion, diced

2 tablespoons minced fresh cilantro leaves

1 radish, thinly sliced

Hot sauce of choice

Preheat the oven to 425°F. Place the tortillas on a baking sheet and evenly brush oil on both sides of each tortilla. Place the tray in the oven for 4 minutes, flip the tortillas, then bake an additional 2 minutes. While the tortillas are still warm, sprinkle with a pinch of salt and allow to completely cool and crisp up.

To a medium mixing bowl, add the beans and avocado, then mash together really well using a fork.

Fold in the artichoke hearts, garlic, lime zest and juice, and pinches of salt, pepper, and everything seasoning. Taste and adjust seasonings to preference.

Spread 2 to 3 tablespoons of the avocado mixture on to your tostada. Top with tomato, onion, cilantro, radish, and hot sauce and enjoy.

I will always be an oats-for-breakfast type of person because their versatility is top tier. You can make stovetop oats, steel-cut oats, overnight oats, savory oats... truly, you are only limited by your imagination. So if maybe you aren't an oats person, ask yourself why. And no, this is not me forcing you to be an oats person! More just wondering if you've tried them in a different way. For example, my favorite suggestion for those who aren't fans of the texture of oatmeal is to bake them. It changes their texture, making them more cakelike versus creamy. This is a fun variation I love to do that transforms them into an upside-down breakfast cake. Just a few simple ingredients, bake, then do the big reveal to show off the impressive fruit topping. And even if I still can't convince you on oats for breakfast, they make for a great fiber-rich snack or a way to impress friends for brunch.

Peach Upside-Down Baked Oatmeal

SERVES 4 TO 6 • PREP TIME: 15 MINUTES • COOKING TIME: 35 MINUTES

1 to 2 ripe peaches (about ½ pound), pitted and thinly sliced into half-moons

1 tablespoon ground flaxseeds

2 ripe bananas

⅓ cup natural almond butter or peanut butter

2 tablespoons agave syrup or maple syrup, or to taste

1 cup unsweetened soy milk or almond milk

2 teaspoons vanilla extract

2 teaspoons baking powder

½ teaspoon kosher salt

2 cups gluten-free rolled oats

Coconut whipped cream, for serving

Preheat the oven to 350°F. Line a 9 × 9 × 2-inch ceramic baking dish with parchment paper.

Layer the peaches to cover the bottom of the baking dish, making sure to fill any gaps, then set aside.

In a small bowl, combine the flaxseeds with 2 tablespoons of water, mix, and set to the side.

To a large mixing bowl, add the bananas, then use a fork to mash them well. Add the flaxseed mixture, nut butter, agave syrup, soy milk, vanilla, baking powder, and salt, then whisk to fully combine.

For a more cakey consistency, place 1 cup of your rolled oats into a food processor and blend for 30 seconds until coarse. Add all the oats to the wet ingredients, then stir well until fully combined. Pour the oat batter over the arranged peaches in the baking dish, then bake in the oven for 35 minutes.

Allow the oatmeal to cool for at least 15 to 20 minutes to fully set. Use a knife to trace along the edge of the baking dish. Top the baking dish with a flat cutting board, then carefully flip to release the oatmeal. Peel away the parchment paper, cut, and serve upside down topped with some coconut whipped cream to make it even more special.

Store leftovers in an airtight container in the fridge for up to 4 days.

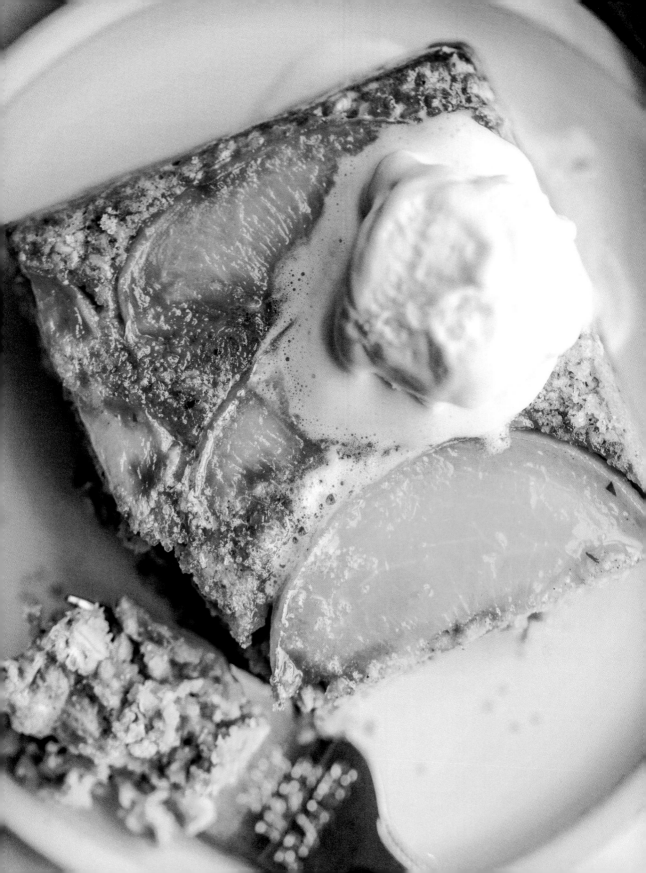

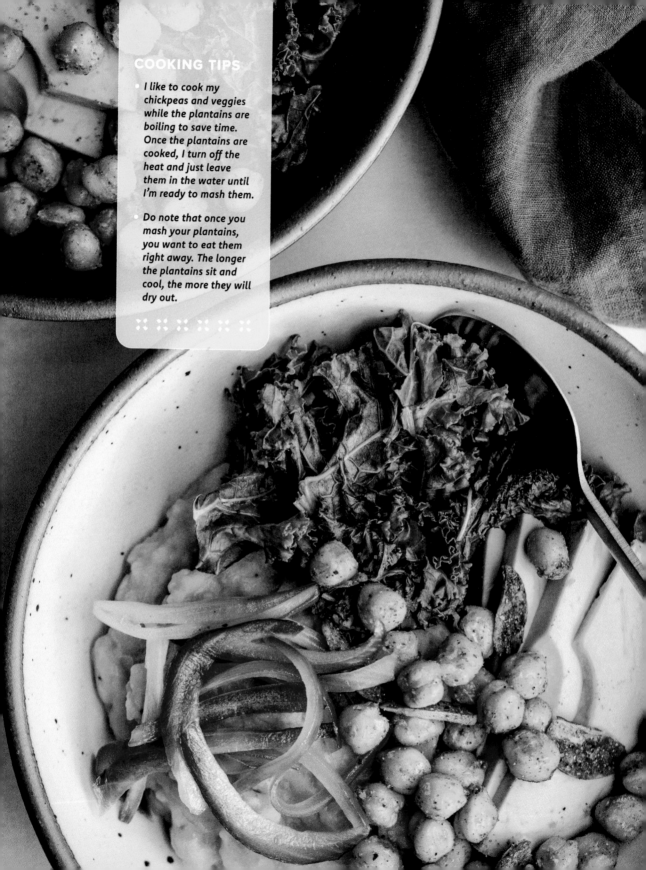

COOKING TIPS

- *I like to cook my chickpeas and veggies while the plantains are boiling to save time. Once the plantains are cooked, I turn off the heat and just leave them in the water until I'm ready to mash them.*

- *Do note that once you mash your plantains, you want to eat them right away. The longer the plantains sit and cool, the more they will dry out.*

I think the hardest part about being a "*no sabo*" kid (Latinos who do not speak fluent Spanish), let alone one who doesn't eat meat, is that sinking feeling like you don't belong anywhere. And whenever I've felt that the most, or felt disconnected from my cultures, cooking familiar foods has always given me the sense of belonging I yearned for. Food gives me an opportunity to reconnect with my culture without having to say a single word. I can enjoy the warm memories I associate with it and just find that familiar feeling of comfort that puts my mind at ease.

Mangú Power Bowl with Crispy Adobo Chickpeas and Onions

SERVES 2 TO 3 • PREP TIME: 15 MINUTES • COOKING TIME: 30 MINUTES

FOR THE CHICKPEAS AND VEGETABLES

1 15-ounce can chickpeas, drained and rinsed

2 tablespoons plus 1 teaspoon avocado oil

½ teaspoon adobo seasoning

½ teaspoon smoked paprika

¼ teaspoon ground coriander

¼ teaspoon dried oregano

Kosher salt to taste

2 garlic cloves, thinly sliced

½ medium red onion, cut into strips

1 tablespoon apple cider vinegar

6 leaves of curly kale, stems removed and roughly chopped

FOR THE MANGÚ

Kosher salt

2 plump green plantains

FOR THE CHICKPEAS AND VEGETABLES

Place your chickpeas on a clean kitchen towel and carefully pat them dry to remove as much excess water as possible.

Warm a nonstick skillet over medium heat, then add 1 tablespoon of the oil. Once the oil is warmed through, add the chickpeas and then top with the adobo, paprika, coriander, oregano, and a pinch of salt. Toss the chickpeas in the spices to evenly coat, then spread the chickpeas out in a single layer and sear undisturbed for 2 minutes. Add the garlic, then give the chickpeas a toss, spread them out again, and sear again for another 2 minutes. Continue to stir the chickpeas occasionally for an extra 3 minutes until they appear blistered and slightly crisp around the edges.

Transfer the chickpeas to a paper towel–lined plate, then add the onion to the pan with a pinch of salt. Sauté the onion for 2 to 3 minutes until it starts to soften. Add the vinegar and continue to cook until the onion starts to turn bright pink in color, then transfer to a plate.

To the same pan, add 1 teaspoon of the oil. Add the kale with a pinch of salt, and sauté until the kale has wilted and turned bright green in color, 2 to 3 minutes.

FOR THE MANGÚ

Bring a large saucepan filled with water to a boil. Once boiling, add a generous pinch of salt to the water.

Recipe continues

Avocado slices

Lime wedges

Hot sauce

Cut the ends of the plantains off. Use a paring knife to cut a slit lengthwise into one of the seams on the skin of the plantain. Use the knife and push the skin apart and remove the peel. If the skin is stubborn, use the knife to help with peeling it away from the flesh. Cut the plantain in half lengthwise, then cut each half in half again lengthwise. Repeat for the second plantain.

Carefully drop the plantains into the boiling water and cook for 12 to 15 minutes or until very tender. Reserve ⅓ cup of the cooking water.

Transfer the cooked plantains to a shallow bowl. Add the remaining 1 tablespoon of oil with a pinch of salt and mash the plantains well with a fork until few lumps remain. Pour in half the reserved plantain water, mixing and mashing to fully incorporate. Stir in the remaining water and continue to mash and mix until mostly smooth, similar to mashed potatoes.

TO SERVE

Serve a portion of the mangú in a bowl and top with the onion. Add the kale and chickpeas on the side, serve with a few slices of avocado, a lime wedge, some hot sauce, and enjoy.

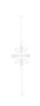

Many people I know have grown up enjoying pancakes made using a classic box mix. The convenience is unmatched, especially for parents trying to make a quick breakfast for hungry young ones. Just measure the dry mix, stir it together with your wet ingredients, and you're ready to make pancakes. I wanted the same convenience, especially considering a lot of pre-packaged pancake mixes contain some dairy in the ingredients, so I made my own. And it works like a charm, plus I can modify it to include things I like. These pancakes have some added wholesomeness to them in the form of hemp hearts and whole grains, but they still manage to be fluffy and tender like the box mixes I remember enjoying on Sunday mornings with my siblings. Just use the amount you need and store the rest for later.

DIY Pancake Mix

MAKES 20 PANCAKES • PREP TIME: 15 MINUTES • COOKING TIME: 20 MINUTES

FOR THE PANCAKE MIX

2 cups (260g) all-purpose flour, spooned and leveled

2 cups (260g) whole wheat pastry flour or more all-purpose flour, spooned and leveled

4 tablespoons (48g) sugar

4 tablespoons (32g) hemp hearts

4 tablespoons (44g) baking powder

1 teaspoon baking soda

1 teaspoon kosher salt

SEE TO MAKE 5 PANCAKES ON PAGE 31

PREPARE THE PANCAKE MIX

To a large mixing bowl, add the flours, sugar, hemp hearts, baking powder, baking soda, and salt. Stir together using a whisk for at least 1 minute to make sure everything is well combined. Transfer the pancake mix to a large airtight container and store in a cool, dry place for up to 1 month.

MAKE 5 PANCAKES

To a large glass measuring cup, add soy milk and vinegar then whisk and allow to sit for 5 minutes. Add the yogurt and vanilla then whisk again until smooth.

Add the pancake mix to a large mixing bowl then pour in the milk mixture. Use a spatula to fold the flour mixture into the wet ingredients until the batter is just combined. Do not overmix the batter! Remove the spatula from the bowl and allow the batter to sit and fluff up while you prepare to cook the pancakes.

Heat a large nonstick pan or griddle for 2 to 3 minutes over medium-low heat. Evenly grease the pan with 1 teaspoon of the oil. When the pan is hot enough, ladle ¼ cup of batter into the pan.

Cook the pancake undisturbed for 2 minutes until the bottom is golden brown in color. You'll know to flip when the edge of the pancake appear to dry out and bubbles form around the center.

Recipe continues

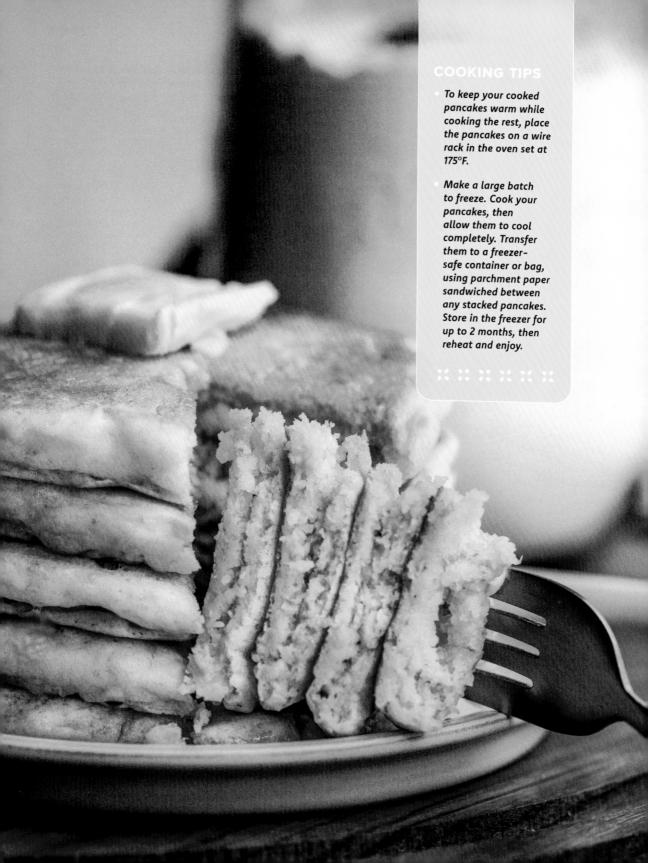

½ cup plus 2 tablespoons unsweetened soy milk

1 tablespoon apple cider vinegar

¼ cup plain unsweetened plant-based yogurt

1 teaspoon vanilla extract

1 cup dry pancake mix, spooned and leveled

1 tablespoon plus 2 teaspoons avocado oil

FOR SERVING

Maple syrup

Fresh jam

Vegan butter

Flip the pancake and cook for 1 minute and 30 seconds. Transfer the cooked pancake to a wire rack, then regrease the pan with another teaspoon of oil and repeat with the remaining batter.

TO SERVE

Serve your pancakes the way you like. Try them with maple syrup, fresh jam, and/or a pat of vegan butter on top and enjoy.

CHAPTER 2

Salads don't just have to be a BORING BOWL of lettuce. These salads are protein packed and LOADED WITH INCREDIBLE FLAVORS and textures that will make you FEEL EXCITED about getting your veggies in.

Satisfying Salads

In the past couple of years, it seems like Brussels sprouts have had their major redemption arc, and I'm here for it! When prepared right, you can get the best flavors and textures out of these sprouts. I love them thinly sliced into shreds, seasoned well, then roasted until slightly caramelized and crispy around the edges. Honestly, I can eat them straight from the pan this way, but I also like to stir them into rice to make a rice salad of sorts. You know, just a fun way to get in more veggies.

Spicy Peanut Shaved Brussels Sprout Salad

SERVES 3 • PREP TIME: 15 MINUTES • COOKING TIME: 25 MINUTES

FOR THE BRUSSELS SPROUTS

1 pound Brussels sprouts, thinly sliced

1 shallot, thinly sliced

1 tablespoon avocado oil

2 teaspoons maple syrup

1 teaspoon garlic powder

¼ teaspoon five-spice powder

Kosher salt and freshly ground black pepper to taste

FOR THE MARINATED SESAME EDAMAME

1½ cups frozen edamame, thawed

1 tablespoon soy sauce

1 teaspoon sesame oil

1 teaspoon rice vinegar

1 garlic clove, grated

Juice of ½ lime

PREPARE THE BRUSSELS SPROUTS

Preheat the oven to 425°F. Line a baking sheet with parchment paper.

To the prepared baking sheet, add the sliced Brussels sprouts and shallot. Drizzle with the oil and maple syrup, then season with the garlic powder, the five-spice powder, and a generous pinch of salt and pepper. Toss to coat, making sure the Brussels sprouts are well-coated, and spread out in a single layer on the baking sheet.

Place the tray in the oven to bake for 15 minutes. Give the Brussels sprouts a toss and return to the oven for 8 to 10 more minutes until the Brussels sprouts are golden around the edges.

PREPARE THE MARINATED SESAME EDAMAME

To a medium mixing bowl, combine the edamame, soy sauce, sesame oil, vinegar, garlic, and lime juice. Toss together to evenly coat and set to the side.

Recipe continues

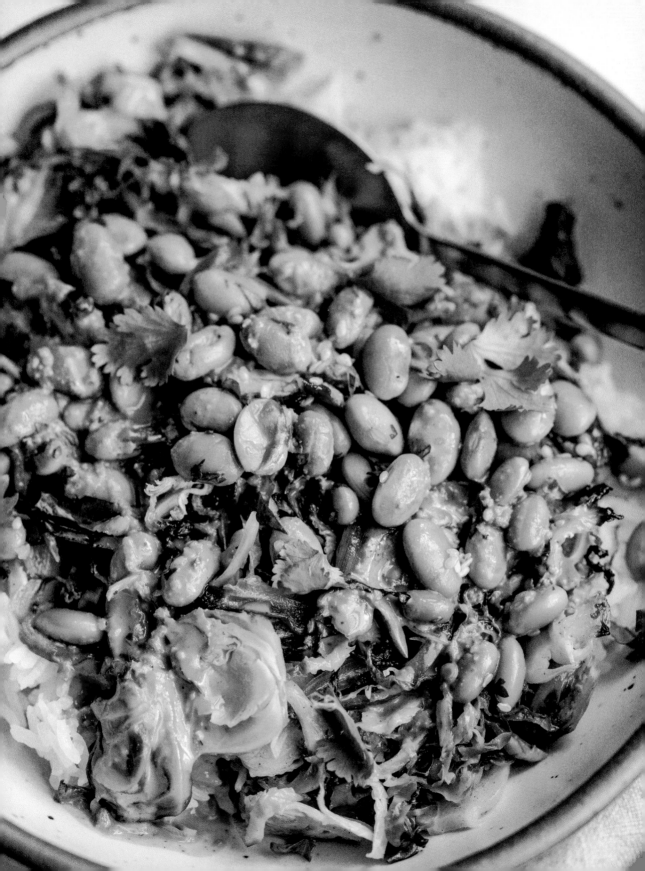

2 cups cooked rice or quinoa
(see page 228)

Chili Crunch Peanut Sauce
(page 215)

1 scallion, thinly sliced

⅓ cup fresh cilantro leaves,
minced

¼ cup salted peanuts,
chopped

TO SERVE

Once the Brussels sprouts are done cooking, mix them into the rice. To
assemble the bowls, serve a portion of the mixed rice and top with a portion of the seasoned edamame. Drizzle with the peanut sauce, then garnish with scallion, cilantro, and chopped peanuts and serve.

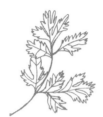

Not all salads need to contain greens. In fact, we're straying away from the expected salad formula and instead utilizing seared poblano peppers and corn to establish our salad base. From here you can add more texture and freshness by including some crispy chickpeas, avocado, and raw red onions. Marry the ingredients together with some lime, garlic, and fresh herbs, and you have the most refreshing and satisfying bowl.

Charred Poblano Corn Salad

SERVES 4 • PREP TIME: 15 MINUTES • COOKING TIME: 30 MINUTES

FOR THE CRISPY ROASTED CHICKPEAS

1 15-ounce can chickpeas, drained and rinsed

1 tablespoon avocado oil

½ teaspoon Old Bay seasoning

Kosher salt to taste

FOR THE POBLANO CORN SALAD

2 poblano peppers

2 ears of corn, shucked

¼ cup red onion, thinly sliced

¼ cup fresh cilantro leaves, minced

¼ cup pepitas

1 garlic clove, finely minced

¼ teaspoon Old Bay seasoning

1 tablespoon red wine vinegar

1 tablespoon extra-virgin olive oil

Zest and juice of 1 lime

Kosher salt and freshly ground black pepper to taste

PREPARE THE CRISPY ROASTED CHICKPEAS

Preheat the oven to 425°F. Line a baking sheet with parchment paper. Place the chickpeas on a clean kitchen towel and carefully pat dry of excess moisture. To the prepared baking sheet, add the chickpeas and drizzle with the avocado oil. Toss to evenly coat, then spread out into a single layer on the sheet. Bake for 20 minutes. Add the Old Bay seasoning and a pinch of salt, then toss to coat using tongs. Place back in the oven for an additional 5 to 10 minutes until crispy.

PREPARE THE POBLANO CORN SALAD

Place a cast-iron skillet or heavy-bottomed pan over medium heat. Once hot, add the whole poblano peppers and corn to the pan and allow to sear undisturbed for 2 minutes. Rotate the peppers and corn every 1 to 2 minutes until all sides are charred, about 10 minutes.

Transfer the poblano peppers to a plastic bag or an airtight container with a lid for 5 minutes. Doing this will allow the pepper to steam and make it easier to remove the skin.

Set the corn aside on a cutting board to cool, and when cool enough to handle, use a knife to cut the corn off the cob and transfer to a large mixing bowl.

Use your hands to peel and discard the skins from the peppers. Cut off the top and remove the stem, then remove the seeds. Dice the peppers, then transfer to the mixing bowl with the corn.

Next, add the onion, cilantro, and pepitas to the bowl.

Recipe continues

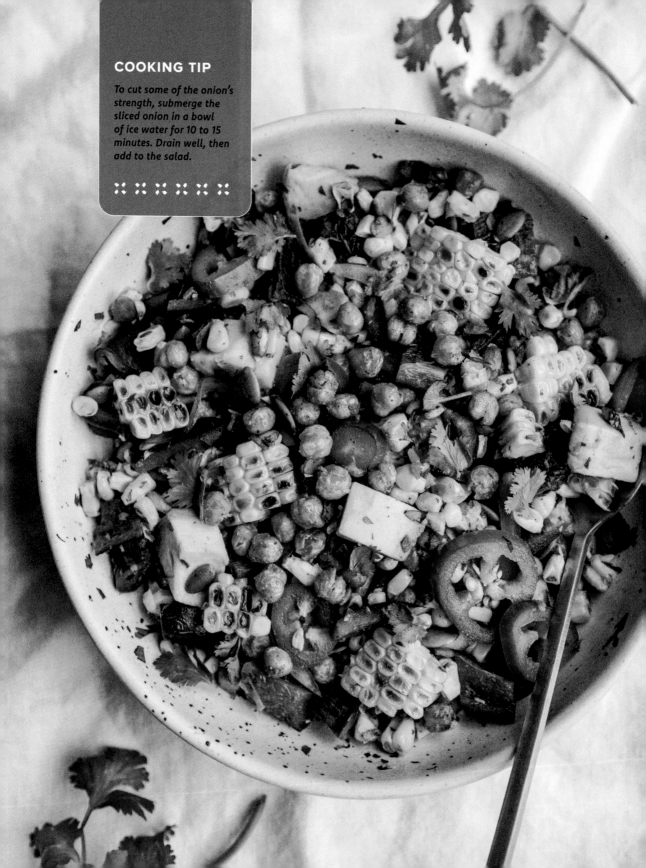

COOKING TIP

To cut some of the onion's strength, submerge the sliced onion in a bowl of ice water for 10 to 15 minutes. Drain well, then add to the salad.

✕ ✕ ✕ ✕ ✕ ✕

1 avocado, cubed

Easy Pickled Jalapeños
(page 171; optional)

In a separate small bowl, whisk together the garlic, Old Bay seasoning, vinegar, olive oil, lime zest and juice, and a pinch of salt and pepper. Pour the dressing over the pepper and corn mixture, then toss together to coat.

TO SERVE

Fold in the cubed avocado. Adjust the salt and pepper to taste, then top with the crispy chickpeas and pickled jalapeños, if desired.

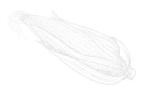

"That's it." Now just imagine saying that with a tone of confusion and then awe. That was exactly how I felt after making these chickpeas. I was amazed by the fact this required so few ingredients, yet had the most incredible taste. Just nine ingredients plus the salt and oil. Now, the magic behind this recipe lies in how you treat your ingredients. Lemon on its own is bright, zingy, and fresh. Lemon that has been charred is a whole different experience and provides a slightly smoky, sweeter flavor. It complements the flavors of the dates and spice from the Fresno chile super well.

Seared Lemon Chickpea Salad

SERVES 3 • PREP TIME: 15 MINUTES • COOKING TIME: 15 MINUTES

1 15-ounce can chickpeas, drained and rinsed

1 garlic clove, grated

1 tablespoon red wine vinegar

1 large lemon

1 tablespoon extra-virgin olive oil

1 shallot, diced

Kosher salt to taste

5 Medjool dates, pits removed and diced

1 Fresno chile, seeded and sliced (optional)

¼ cup fresh parsley, minced

5 fresh mint leaves, minced

Add the chickpeas to a medium mixing bowl and top with the garlic. Then pour the vinegar over the garlic to help mellow out the flavor.

Zest the whole lemon over the chickpeas, then cut the lemon in half.

Heat up a medium skillet with half the oil over medium-low heat. When the oil is hot, place both lemon halves face side down into the oil and allow to sear for 4 to 5 minutes undisturbed until the bottoms appear nicely charred.

Remove the lemons carefully with tongs, then place the lemons in a lemon squeezer and squeeze the juice on top of the chickpeas (if squeezing with your hands, make sure your hands are clean and that the lemons have had a few moments to cool before handling).

Add the remaining oil to the same skillet and add the shallot with a pinch of salt. Sauté until the shallot has softened, about 2 minutes.

Stir in the dates and chile (if using) and continue to sauté until they are warmed through, about 3 minutes, and remove from heat.

Add the date mixture to the bowl of chickpeas along with the parsley, mint, and a generous pinch of salt. Give the mixture a good toss to fully combine, then taste and adjust the salt to your liking.

Allow the chickpeas to marinate in the fridge for at least 30 minutes before enjoying.

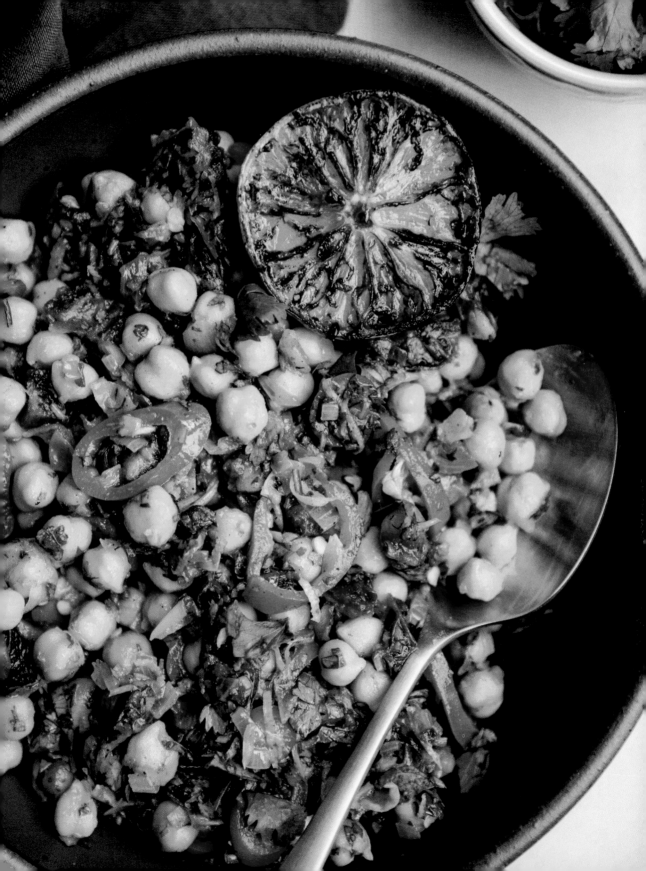

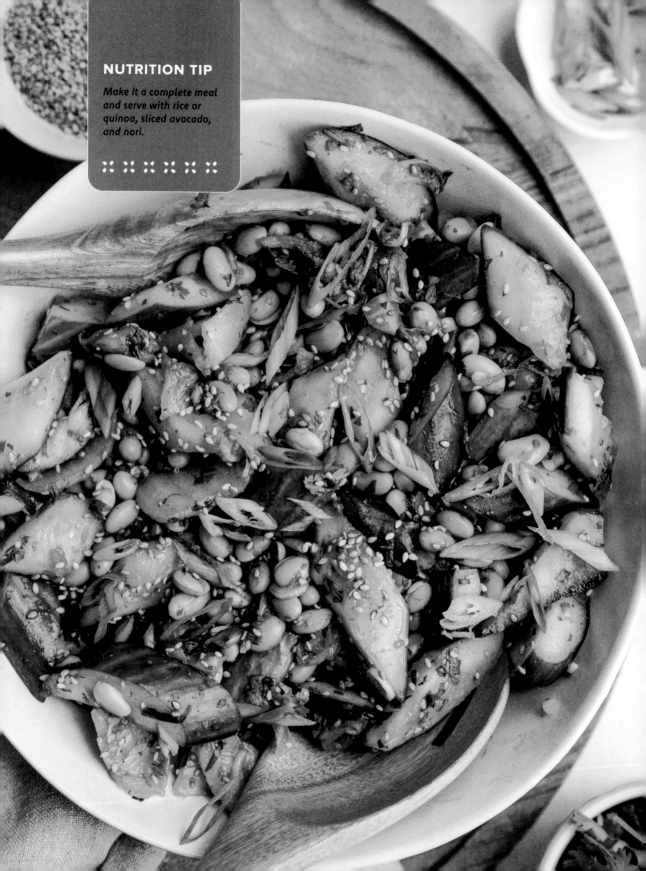

NUTRITION TIP

Make it a complete meal and serve with rice or quinoa, sliced avocado, and nori.

I joke a lot and say that when I'm frustrated, you will find me in the kitchen making a cucumber salad. And I say this because we aren't just chopping up a cucumber for it, we are smashing the cucumber. If you are not familiar with this Chinese technique, you use the flat of your knife to smash the cucumbers, which helps release water and creates more surface area for flavor to get in. It also just happens to be a productive way of getting some frustrations out.

Smashed Cucumber Kimchi Edamame Salad

SERVES 3 • PREP TIME: 25 MINUTES

2 English cucumbers

Kosher salt to taste

Sugar

1 tablespoon gochujang

1 garlic clove, grated

1 tablespoon toasted sesame oil

2 tablespoons soy sauce

Zest and juice of 1 lime

1 to 2 teaspoons maple syrup

2 cups frozen edamame, thawed

¼ cup vegan kimchi, chopped

3 tablespoons minced fresh cilantro leaves

2 scallions, thinly sliced

1 tablespoon toasted sesame seeds

Cut the ends off the cucumbers, then cut them in half lengthwise. Place your halved cucumbers cut side down on the cutting board and, with the flat side of your knife, smack down along the length of the cucumbers until they split. Slice the smashed cucumbers diagonally into ½-inch pieces.

Transfer the cut cucumbers to a sieve propped on top of a medium bowl. Top the cucumbers with a generous sprinkle of salt and sugar and allow to sit and drain for 20 minutes.

While the cucumbers drain, prepare your sauce. To a large mixing bowl, add the gochujang, garlic, sesame oil, soy sauce, lime zest and juice, and maple syrup, then whisk together until smooth.

Give the cucumbers a gentle squeeze to release a little additional liquid, then discard the excess water. Do not rinse the cucumbers! Place the cucumbers into the bowl with the dressing along with the edamame, kimchi, cilantro, scallions, and sesame seeds.

Toss everything together to combine, then serve immediately or allow to marinate in the fridge. Leftovers can be stored in an airtight container in the fridge for up to 5 days.

When I was interning and on my way to becoming a dietitian, one of my nutrition rotations had me travel to an industrial building where we had to try and convince a group of factory workers to be enthusiastic about eating vegetables—and let's just say it wasn't easy. Regardless of the health and preventative benefits we shared, they didn't really care, and I don't blame them for that. People are inundated with nutrition information all the time, and it will only matter to someone if what you are sharing can fit in their lives. And the thing that made the biggest impact was actually giving them examples of how you could make vegetables taste so much better than expected. So I worked on a handout and then one night I spent time massaging kale in a simple dressing to help soften it to improve its taste and texture. I set up all my hard work in their break room and everyone was skeptical when they looked at it. A few brave people decided to give it a try, which then caused more people to try it. Even the pickiest of the group was surprised that they actually liked kale this way, let alone at all. Since then, I've made many variations of this salad. This one uses white beans and hemp hearts to add protein and is then massaged with an umami-rich tahini dressing to make it super satisfying.

Creamy Lemon Miso Chopped Kale Salad

SERVES 3 • PREP TIME: 15 MINUTES

6 cups kale, stems removed, chopped

Zest and juice of 1 lemon

1 teaspoon toasted sesame oil

Kosher salt to taste

2 tablespoons hemp hearts

2 scallions, thinly sliced

1 garlic clove, grated

3 tablespoons good-quality tahini (see page 59)

2 teaspoons yellow or white miso paste

2 teaspoons maple syrup

1 15-ounce can cannellini beans, drained and rinsed

1 avocado, sliced

Freshly ground black pepper

To a large mixing bowl, add the chopped kale and top with the lemon zest, sesame oil, and a generous pinch of salt. Use your hands to rub the zest and salt into the greens until the kale has shrunk in size and become softer in texture, about 2 minutes.

To the kale, add the hemp hearts and scallions, then set the bowl aside to make the dressing.

To a separate small mixing bowl, add the garlic, lemon juice, tahini, miso paste, and maple syrup, then whisk together until completely smooth. As you mix, you may notice the sauce thicken. To thin it out, add 1 tablespoon of cold water at a time while whisking until you reach your desired consistency.

Pour half the dressing over the bowl of kale and toss to evenly combine.

Add the beans and avocado along with the remaining dressing, season with a pinch of pepper, and carefully fold everything together. Adjust salt and pepper to taste and enjoy.

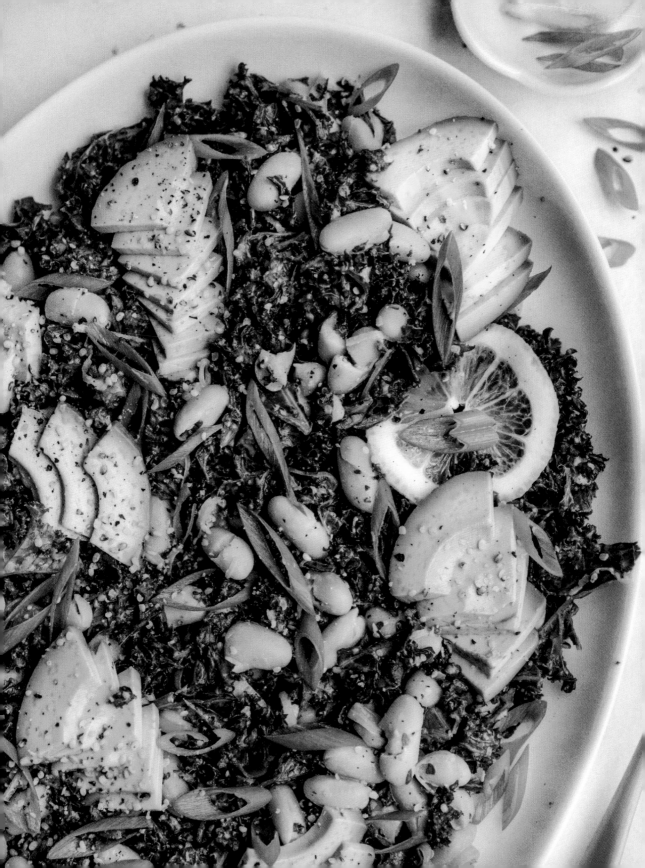

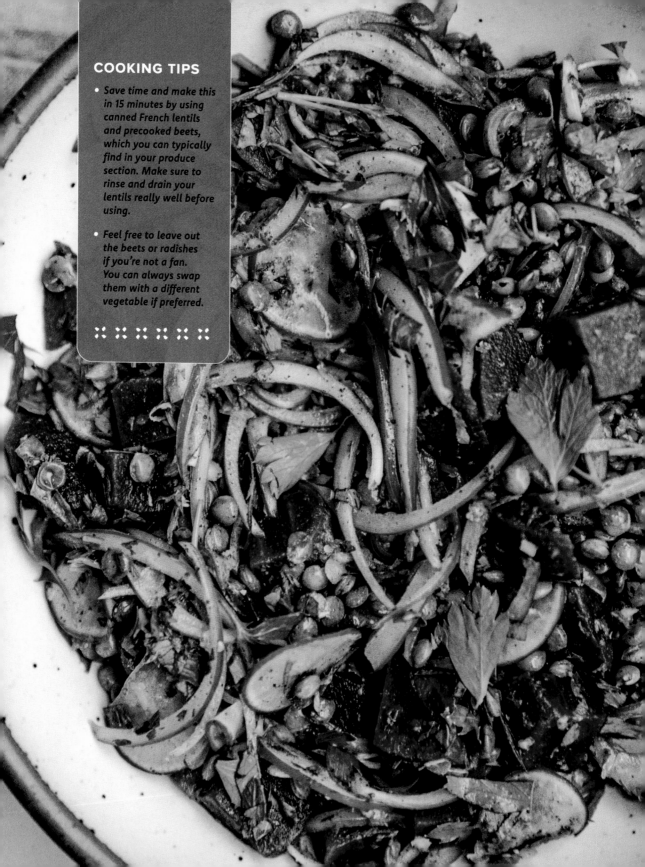

COOKING TIPS

- Save time and make this in 15 minutes by using canned French lentils and precooked beets, which you can typically find in your produce section. Make sure to rinse and drain your lentils really well before using.

- Feel free to leave out the beets or radishes if you're not a fan. You can always swap them with a different vegetable if preferred.

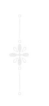

Like many individuals, I am not the biggest fan of raw onions, but if you marinate them in citrus, sumac, and herbs, you can transform their flavor into something truly epic. Toss them together with some high-protein lentils and you have a very satisfying, zingy salad. These marinated onions are inspired by a tangy Turkish onion salad, which is commonly enjoyed along with rich meat dishes like kebab. The addition of sumac adds some complex acidity with a hint of fruitiness that helps balance the harshness of the onions. Honestly, it amazes me how few ingredients you need for this because the blend of flavors here is incredible.

Marinated Sumac Onion and Lentil Salad

SERVES 3 • PREP TIME: 15 MINUTES • COOKING TIME: 45 MINUTES

1 large beet

1 cup dried French lentils, rinsed well

½ medium red onion, thinly sliced

Kosher salt to taste

1 teaspoon sumac

1 garlic clove, grated

Zest and juice of 1 lemon

⅓ cup fresh parsley, woody stems removed, minced

2 tablespoons extra-virgin olive oil

1 tablespoon maple syrup

1 tablespoon red wine vinegar

4 to 5 radishes, thinly sliced

Warm pita and hummus, for serving

Preheat your oven to 400°F.

Scrub the beet well under warm water, then trim off the base and tip. No need to peel your beet yet. Rub a small amount of oil over the beet, then wrap it tightly in foil. Place the beet on a baking sheet and roast for 45 minutes or until fork-tender. Allow the beet to cool for 15 minutes, then run it under cold water to help remove the skin. Pat the beet dry, then cube it.

While the beets roast, cook your lentils according to package instructions. Once cooked, drain your lentils well and allow to cool.

To a large mixing bowl, add the onion, a pinch of salt, sumac, garlic, lemon zest, half the lemon juice, parsley, and 1 tablespoon of the oil. Stir to combine and allow to marinate in the fridge for at least 15 minutes while preparing the other ingredients.

When ready to mix, add the lentils, beets, maple syrup, vinegar, remaining lemon juice, remaining tablespoon of the oil, radishes, and a generous pinch of salt. Toss everything to combine, taste and adjust salt to preference. This salad can be enjoyed served with warm pita and hummus.

Crunchy vegetables mixed with one of my favorite grains, farro—it's the salad I love to make when it starts getting a little cooler outside. It also comes in clutch when I need a yummy way to get my cruciferous vegetables in. Cruciferous vegetables include vegetables like bok choy, broccoli, Brussels sprouts, cabbage, cauliflower, and kale. They are rich in vitamin C and E, good sources of fiber, and packed with sulfur-containing components that may help with lowering inflammation and reducing the risk of chronic diseases such as cancer. Sulfur also happens to be a component of what can make these veggies have a bitter taste to them. To help combat that, we balance the flavors by caramelizing the veggies in the oven and complementing them with a sweet citrusy sauce.

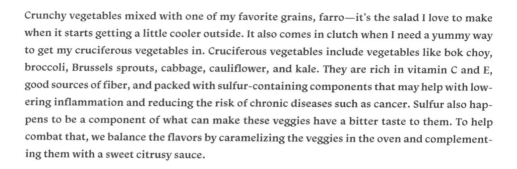

Roasted Cruciferous Crunch Salad

SERVES 3 • PREP TIME: 15 MINUTES • COOKING TIME: 15 MINUTES

2 cups green cabbage, shredded

1 cup red cabbage, shredded

½ red onion, thinly sliced

2 cups broccoli florets, cut into bite-size pieces

2 tablespoons avocado oil, plus more as needed

1 teaspoon onion powder

1 teaspoon garlic powder

1 teaspoon five-spice powder

Kosher salt to taste

1 8-ounce block of tempeh

1 tablespoon soy sauce

1 tablespoon mirin

2 teaspoons maple syrup

Zest and juice of ½ lime

1 cup cooked farro (see page 228), to serve

Orange Ginger Tahini Dressing (page 210), to serve

Fresh cilantro leaves, to serve

Sesame seeds, to serve

Preheat the oven to 400°F. Line 2 baking sheets with parchment paper.

To the prepared baking sheet, add the green and red cabbage, red onion, and broccoli. Drizzle the vegetables with at least 1 tablespoon of oil, then add the onion powder, garlic powder, ½ teaspoon five-spice powder, and a generous pinch of salt. Massage the spices and oil into the vegetables until well coated (use more oil as needed). Spread the vegetables out on the baking sheet into a single layer. If the vegetables are overlapping, use a second tray to give the vegetables more space.

On a different prepared baking sheet, use your hands to crumble the tempeh into very small pieces. Drizzle with the soy sauce, mirin, and remaining 1 tablespoon of the oil, then toss together to combine and spread out on the tray in a single layer.

Place the vegetable tray on the top rack of the oven and the tempeh on the bottom rack, then bake for 15 to 17 minutes, tossing halfway. The vegetables and tempeh should look slightly charred around the edges.

Once the vegetables and tempeh come out of the oven, add the maple syrup and lime zest and juice to the tempeh and toss to coat.

To assemble your bowl, add a serving of farro, top with a portion of the roasted cabbage and broccoli. Top with the crispy tempeh then drizzle on the Orange Ginger Tahini Dressing and garnish with cilantro and sesame seeds.

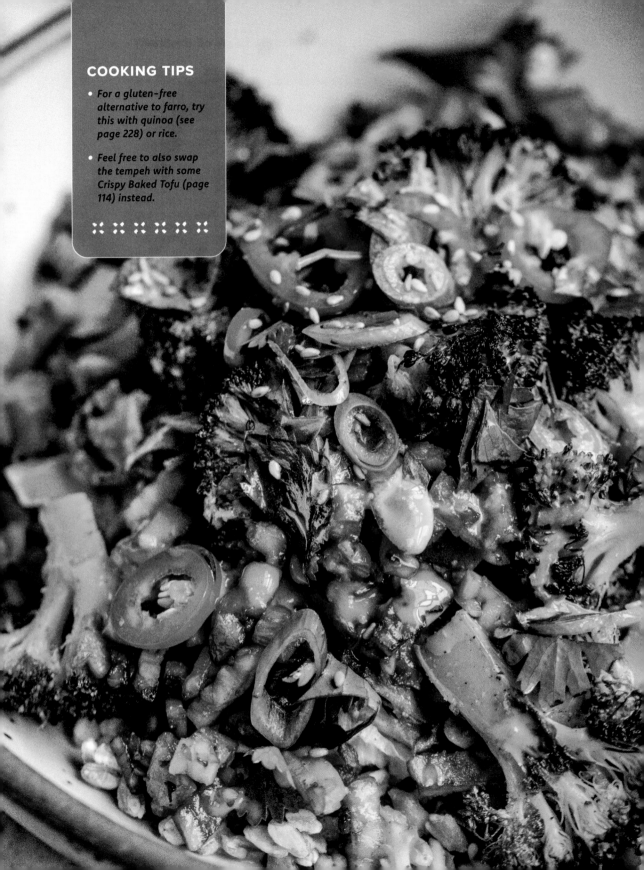

COOKING TIPS

- For a gluten-free alternative to farro, try this with quinoa (see page 228) or rice.

- Feel free to also swap the tempeh with some Crispy Baked Tofu (page 114) instead.

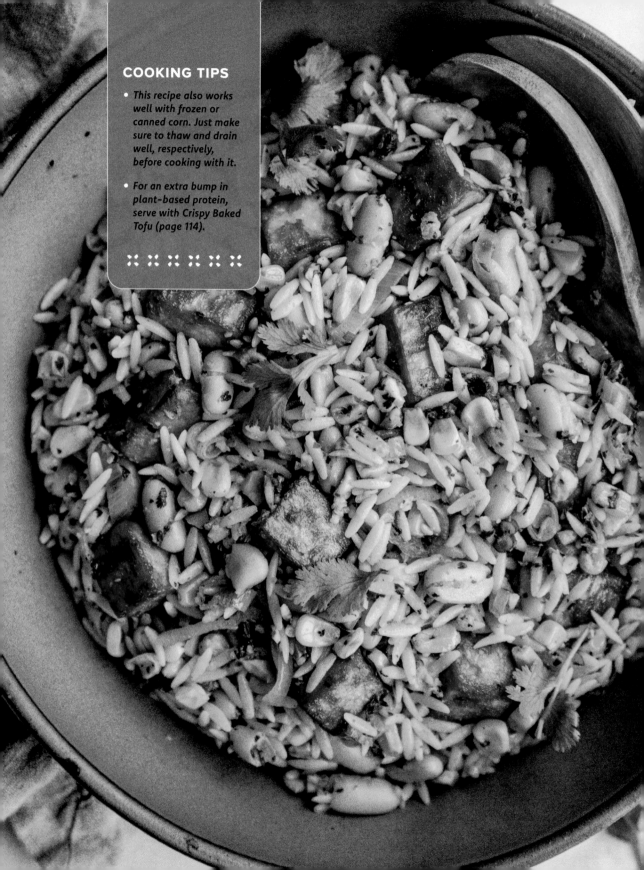

COOKING TIPS

- This recipe also works well with frozen or canned corn. Just make sure to thaw and drain well, respectively, before cooking with it.

- For an extra bump in plant-based protein, serve with Crispy Baked Tofu (page 114).

I am very particular about pasta salads. Honestly, the only way I'll eat them is if they are of the orzo kind. This variation tosses orzo together with some fresh seared corn that has been infused with cumin seeds and garlic. I would happily eat this as is, but paired with the cilantro lime dressing it truly completes the dish and gives it the right amount of freshness and tangy goodness. So if you struggle with pasta salad, too, this one might change your mind.

Pistachio Lime Corn Orzo Salad

SERVES 4 • PREP TIME: 10 MINUTES • COOKING TIME: 20 MINUTES

FOR THE ORZO SALAD

Kosher salt to taste

1 cup orzo

1 tablespoon extra-virgin olive oil

1 teaspoon cumin seeds

1 large shallot, sliced

2 ears of corn, shucked and kernels removed from the cobs

3 garlic cloves, crushed with a garlic press

½ teaspoon ground coriander

2 scallions, thinly sliced

1 15-ounce can cannellini beans, drained and rinsed

¼ cup jarred sun-dried tomatoes packed in oil, sliced

⅓ cup chopped pistachios or pepitas (optional)

PREPARE THE ORZO SALAD

Bring a large saucepan full of water to a boil over high heat. Salt it generously, then once back to a boil, add the orzo and cook for 9 minutes until al dente, stirring occasionally to prevent the pasta from sticking to the bottom of the pan. Drain the orzo (do not rinse) and place in a large mixing bowl.

While the orzo is cooking, place a large skillet over medium-low heat and add the oil. Once the oil is hot, add the cumin seeds and toast for about 1 minute. Add the shallot with a pinch of salt and sauté until softened, about 2 minutes.

Stir in the corn, then spread the mixture out and allow to cook undisturbed for 2 to 3 minutes. Add the garlic and coriander, then continue to sauté for 2 minutes until fragrant.

Transfer the corn mixture to the bowl with the orzo and add the scallions, beans, sun-dried tomatoes, and pistachios or pepitas, if using.

Recipe continues

1 cup packed fresh cilantro
leaves

1 jalapeño, seeded and
roughly chopped

1 garlic clove, grated

Zest and juice of 2 limes

¼ cup extra-virgin olive oil

1 tablespoon maple syrup

½ teaspoon kosher salt

PREPARE THE CILANTRO LIME DRESSING

To a small food processor cup, add the cilantro, jalapeño, garlic, lime zest and juice, oil, maple syrup, and salt, then blitz together until the ingredients are finely minced. Pour the dressing over the orzo, then toss to combine. Adjust salt to taste, then enjoy.

My secret to crispy sweet potatoes? A little cornstarch. When mixed with the oil and coated on the sweet potatoes, it will absorb some excess moisture, and you are left with a crispy exterior with a nice tender inside. These sweet potatoes are fantastic on top of salads like this one. Again, we are adding flavor and different textures to every layer of this salad. You get crispy chickpeas and sweet potato, charred and tender cauliflower, and fluffy quinoa in each bite. Don't forget the cooling and tangy yogurt sauce. That is a must to help balance all the yummy flavors here.

Smoky Roasted Sweet Potato Quinoa Salad

SERVES 3 • PREP TIME: 20 MINUTES • COOKING TIME: 35 MINUTES

FOR THE QUINOA SALAD

1 cup quinoa, rinsed

1 3/4 cups vegetable broth

1 medium sweet potato, peeled and cubed

1 tablespoon cornstarch

2 teaspoons smoked paprika

2 teaspoons garlic powder

1 teaspoon ground coriander

Kosher salt to taste

4 tablespoons avocado oil

2 cups cauliflower, cut into bite-size pieces

1 15-ounce can chickpeas, drained and rinsed

PREPARE THE QUINOA SALAD

Preheat the oven to 425°F. Line 2 baking sheets with parchment paper.

To a medium saucepan, add the quinoa and vegetable broth. Bring to a boil over medium-high heat, then reduce to a simmer and cover with a lid. Allow the quinoa to simmer for 15 minutes. Remove from the heat and allow to stand covered for 10 minutes, then fluff with a fork.

Add the sweet potato pieces to a large resealable bag with the cornstarch, 1 teaspoon paprika, 1 teaspoon garlic powder, ½ teaspoon coriander, and a pinch of salt. Drizzle 1½ tablespoons of oil on top then seal the bag and toss to evenly coat. Spread the potatoes out on one half of one of the prepared baking sheets, leaving space between the potatoes for roasting.

To the same bag, add the cauliflower with 1½ tablespoons oil and the remaining paprika, garlic powder, coriander, and a pinch of salt. Toss to evenly coat, then spread the cauliflower out in a single layer on the other half of the baking sheet opposite the sweet potatoes, placing the florets cut side down on the tray.

Place the chickpeas on a clean kitchen towel and pat dry. Add the chickpeas to the other prepared baking sheet with the remaining tablespoon of oil and a pinch of salt. Toss to evenly coat the chickpeas, then spread them out on the tray in a single layer.

Place both trays in the oven for 30 to 35 minutes, making sure to toss the chickpeas and the potatoes every 10 minutes to help them evenly roast. Give the cauliflower a toss after 20 minutes of roasting.

Recipe continues

½ cup plain unsweetened
plant-based yogurt (thick
consistency preferred)

1 garlic clove, grated or
crushed with a garlic press

Zest and juice of ½ lemon

2 tablespoons fresh
minced dill

Kosher salt to taste

FOR SERVING

Fresh cilantro or parsley
leaves

Pickled Red Onions
(page 172)

PREPARE THE SIMPLE GARLIC YOGURT SAUCE

Once everything is done roasting, place in a small bowl the yogurt, garlic, lemon zest and juice, dill, and a generous pinch of salt, then whisk to combine.

TO SERVE

Add a portion of quinoa to a bowl with a third of the chickpeas, potatoes, and cauliflower. Toss to combine, then top with a drizzle of the dressing and garnish with fresh herbs and pickled onions if you'd like.

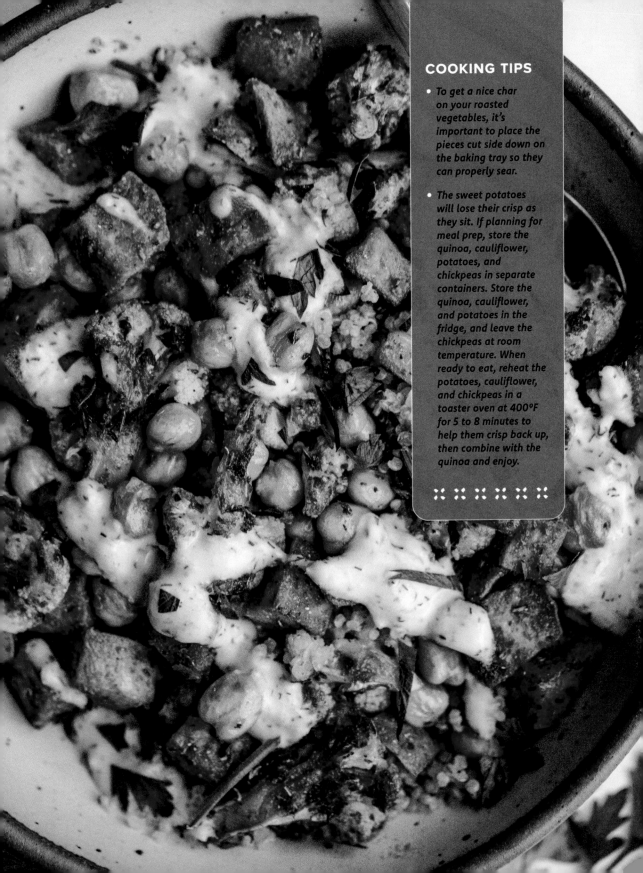

COOKING TIPS

- To get a nice char on your roasted vegetables, it's important to place the pieces cut side down on the baking tray so they can properly sear.

- The sweet potatoes will lose their crisp as they sit. If planning for meal prep, store the quinoa, cauliflower, potatoes, and chickpeas in separate containers. Store the quinoa, cauliflower, and potatoes in the fridge, and leave the chickpeas at room temperature. When ready to eat, reheat the potatoes, cauliflower, and chickpeas in a toaster oven at 400°F for 5 to 8 minutes to help them crisp back up, then combine with the quinoa and enjoy.

CHAPTER 3

It's hard not to be in a rush these days. Regardless of how BUSY YOU ARE, it shouldn't mean that you can't enjoy a NOURISHING meal. These recipes can be prepped with MINIMAL EFFORT for the workweek and stay nice and fresh until you are READY TO EAT. Grab them from the fridge before you leave, and YOU ARE SET for the day.

Grab It & Go

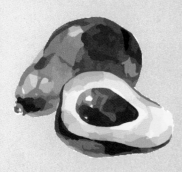

Salads are great, but when you can stuff them into a burrito, even better. This Caesar Salad Wrap does just that and also manages to pack in more plant-based protein by including some seasoned tofu croutons. Not to mention, each component of this wrap also helps you get in a good amount of calcium, too.

Kale Caesar Salad Wrap

SERVES 3 • PREP TIME: 15 MINUTES • COOKING TIME: 35 MINUTES

FOR THE TOFU CROUTONS

1 16-ounce block extra-firm tofu, drained and pressed (see page xxxix)

1 tablespoon cornstarch

1 tablespoon nutritional yeast

2 tablespoons reduced-sodium soy sauce

1½ tablespoons avocado oil

1 teaspoon garlic powder

1 teaspoon onion powder

1 teaspoon Italian seasoning

SEE CREAMY TAHINI CAESAR DRESSING ON PAGE 60

PREPARE THE TOFU CROUTONS

Preheat the oven to 425°F and line a baking sheet with parchment paper.

Pat the tofu dry, cut the tofu into small cubes, and place in a large airtight container. Add the cornstarch, nutritional yeast, soy sauce, oil, garlic powder, onion powder, and Italian seasoning to the container, seal well, and gently shake to evenly coat the tofu. Place the tofu on the prepared baking sheet in a single layer with space between the tofu cubes. Place the tray in the oven for 20 minutes, flip the tofu, and bake for an extra 10 minutes until golden.

PREPARE THE CREAMY TAHINI CAESAR DRESSING

To a small bowl, add the tahini, garlic, lemon zest and juice, capers and caper juice, mustard, miso paste, nutritional yeast, water, a generous pinch of salt, and a pinch of pepper, and whisk until smooth and creamy. If the dressing is too thick, add additional water 1 tablespoon at a time until the dressing is at your desired consistency, adjusting salt to taste as needed.

Chop the kale into bite-size pieces and place in a large mixing bowl. Drizzle the dressing over the kale and massage the dressing into the kale greens until the kale begins to soften and shrink.

Recipe continues

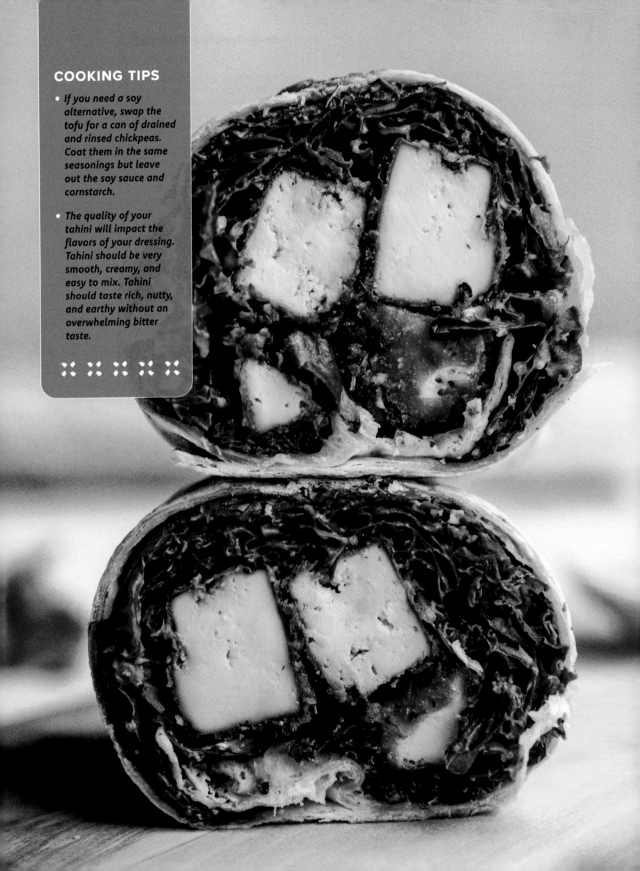

⅓ cup good-quality tahini
(see Cooking Tips)

1 garlic clove, grated or
crushed with a garlic press

Zest and juice of ½ medium
lemon

2 teaspoons capers, finely
minced plus 2 tablespoons
of brine from the caper jar

1 teaspoon Dijon mustard

1 teaspoon yellow or white
miso paste

3 tablespoons nutritional yeast

¼ cup cold water

Kosher salt and freshly ground
black pepper to taste

8 stems of kale, tough stems
removed

TO ASSEMBLE

3 large burrito wraps or tortillas

TO ASSEMBLE

Warm a large tortilla in a dry skillet for 15 seconds on each side. Place the tortilla on a flat surface and fill it with the kale and a handful of tofu croutons. Tuck in the corners of the wrap, fold over, and roll into a tight log.

Heat a medium skillet over medium heat and place the wraps seam-side down and cook for 2 minutes on each side or until the bottom is golden and crispy. Remove from heat and enjoy immediately.

This is dedicated to all the sandwiches and wraps I've ordered out that left me feeling hungry. In the past, a lot of the vegan options available at restaurants didn't always include a significant amount of protein. We're talking veggie tacos with no beans, mushroom wraps, and veggie hummus sandwiches with the tiniest smear of hummus. This wrap, plus others in this book, would be an example of what I'd have available in my hypothetical café. Now, the protein here is in the form of smoky chipotle tofu deli slices. You can easily prep these slices in advance to use in sandwiches and wraps throughout the week. So, stuff your wrap the way you like it, then stuff your face lovingly.

Smoky Chipotle Tofu Wrap

SERVES 4 • PREP TIME: 20 MINUTES • COOKING TIME: 16 MINUTES

FOR THE SMOKY TOFU DELI SLICES

1 16-ounce block super-firm high-protein or extra-firm tofu, drained and pressed (see page 122)

½ teaspoon vegetable bouillon paste or ½ vegetable bouillon cube, crushed

3 tablespoons adobo sauce from a can of chipotle peppers

2 tablespoons maple syrup

1 tablespoon tamari

1 tablespoon apple cider vinegar

1 tablespoon avocado oil

1 teaspoon smoked paprika

½ teaspoon ground coriander

Pinch of white pepper

PREPARE THE SMOKY TOFU DELI SLICES

Preheat the oven to 400°F. Line a baking sheet with parchment paper.

Pat the tofu dry, then place it on a cutting board. Use a sharp knife to cut the tofu block crosswise into thin ⅛-inch slabs (1 to 2 millimeters). Place the slabs on the prepared baking sheet.

To a small bowl, add the bouillon paste and adobo sauce, then stir together until smooth. (If using a bouillon cube, crush up the cube and use a spoon to lightly mash the cube into the sauce until no lumps remain.) Add the maple syrup, tamari, vinegar, oil, smoked paprika, coriander, and pepper, then whisk together until completely smooth and set aside.

Brush to coat the top of each tofu slice with the sauce, then place the tofu in the oven to bake for 8 minutes.

Carefully flip the tofu slices with tongs, then brush the top side with the sauce again. Set the sauce bowl to the side and place the tray back in the oven for 7 to 8 minutes or until the edges start to brown slightly.

Recipe continues

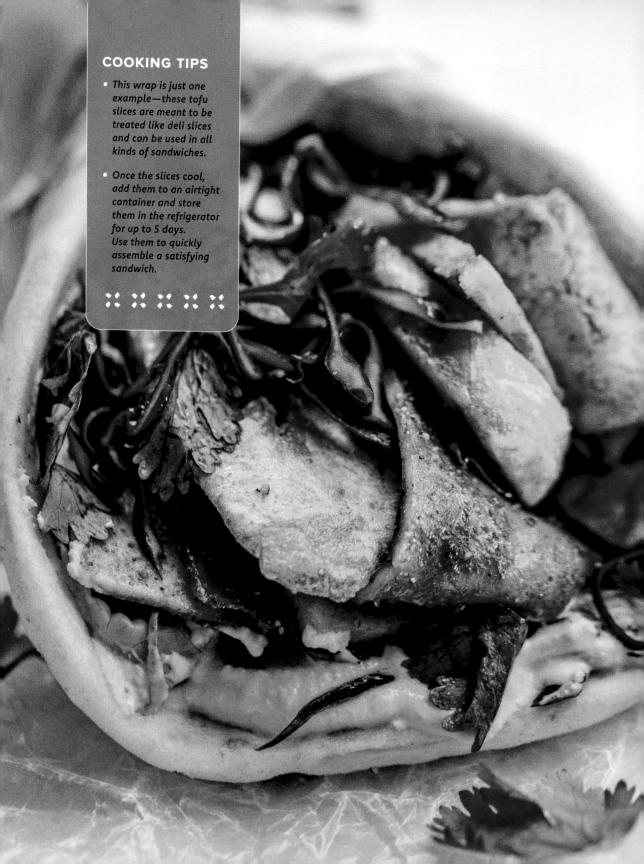

1 cup red cabbage, shredded

2 tablespoons minced fresh
cilantro leaves

1 teaspoon extra-virgin olive oil

1 teaspoon apple cider vinegar

Kosher salt to taste

4 pitas

Jalapeño Lime Crema
(page 219)

Baked Plátanos Maduros
(page 199) or plantain chips
(optional)

PREPARE THE SLAW

While the tofu bakes, in a small bowl, combine the cabbage, cilantro, oil, vinegar, and a pinch of salt. Use clean hands to massage everything together and soften the cabbage.

TO ASSEMBLE THE WRAP AS SHOWN

Warm up the pita in a preheated medium sauté pan over medium-low heat for a few seconds on both sides. Spread each pita with 2 tablespoons or more of crema, then top with a few slices of tofu, 2 slices of plantain, and the cabbage mixture. Wrap it up and enjoy.

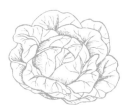

When I think about a quick lunch, my thoughts instantly go to chickpea salad. It's one of the easiest sandwich fillings you can make and one of the most versatile to flavor. So instead of meal prepping the typical spread, I love making this peanut-miso version. It's full of umami flavor thanks to the miso paste, and the peanut butter adds this delicious savory element that helps balance out the sriracha and vinegar blended in, too. Just mash everything up in an airtight container and store in the fridge. When you're ready to eat, just spread it on your favorite bread and load it up with your favorite sandwich fixings. Ta-da, lunch is served!

Peanut Miso Chickpea Salad Sandwich

SERVES 3 • PREP TIME: 10 MINUTES

1 15-ounce can chickpeas, drained and rinsed

2 teaspoons yellow or white miso paste

2 scallions, thinly sliced

1 garlic clove, grated

2 tablespoons salted natural peanut butter

1 tablespoon sriracha

2 teaspoons maple syrup

2 teaspoons rice vinegar

6 to 8 slices of sourdough or whole wheat bread

Sandwich fixings of choice: romaine or leaf lettuce, green or red cabbage, sliced tomatoes, sliced cucumbers, sprouts, cilantro, black sesame seeds, mustard, vegan mayonnaise

To a medium airtight container, add your chickpeas and miso paste, then use a fork to mash them together. When mashing, mash as much of the chickpeas as you personally like. I tend to mash about 2/3 of the chickpeas and leave some whole chickpeas for texture.

Add the scallions, garlic, peanut butter, sriracha, maple syrup, and vinegar, then stir together well to combine. Refrigerate until ready to enjoy. This mixture can be stored in the fridge for up to 4 days.

To assemble a sandwich, add a few spoons of the peanut-miso chickpeas onto a slice of bread and spread it out evenly. Layer on your preferred sandwich fixings, then top with another slice of bread that you can spread with mustard or your favorite vegan mayo. Serve and enjoy!

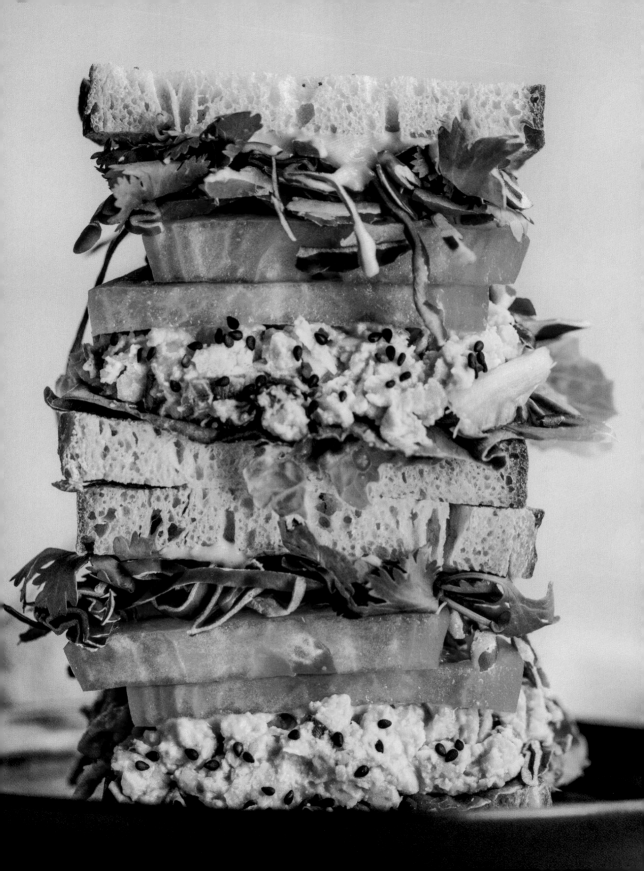

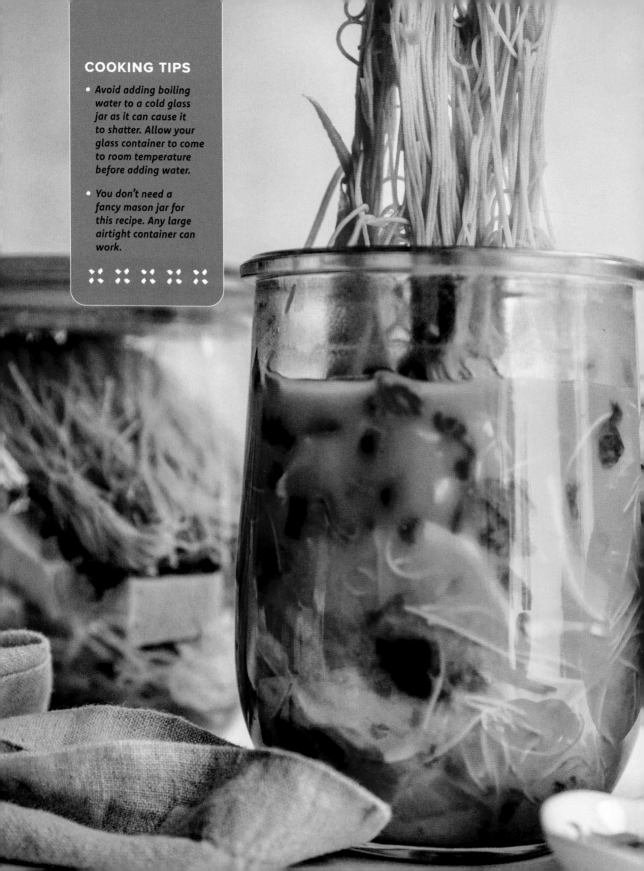

COOKING TIPS

- Avoid adding boiling water to a cold glass jar as it can cause it to shatter. Allow your glass container to come to room temperature before adding water.

- You don't need a fancy mason jar for this recipe. Any large airtight container can work.

Instant noodles were a childhood staple of mine, and if it were up to me, they would have been an everyday meal, too. However, I've moved past that... slightly. And what I mean by that is that I still love noodles, but I also love being able to customize my meals and make them more satisfying. So instead of relying on the typical instant cup noodles, I like to meal prep these Kimchi Noodle Soup Jars instead. They are packed with fresh veggies, noodles, protein, and a delicious gochujang-broth base. Load up your jar exactly the way you like it, and when you're ready to enjoy, just pour over some boiling water.

Kimchi Noodle Soup Jar

SERVES 1 • PREP TIME: 10 MINUTES • COOKING TIME: 5 MINUTES

1 tablespoon gochujang (use less if sensitive to spice)

1 teaspoon toasted sesame oil

1 tablespoon reduced-sodium soy sauce

½ teaspoon vegetable bouillon paste or ½ vegetable bouillon cube, crushed

1 tablespoon salted natural peanut butter

2 tablespoons kimchi, plus 1 tablespoon of the kimchi brine

½ cup shredded green or red cabbage

¼ cup shredded carrots

1 spring onion, thinly sliced

3 ounces extra-firm tofu, drained, pressed (see page xxxix), and cubed

2 tablespoons roughly chopped fresh cilantro leaves

1 bundle vermicelli rice noodles

Into the bottom of a 1-liter jar, place the gochujang, sesame oil, soy sauce, vegetable bouillon paste, peanut butter, and kimchi brine.

Give the mixture a good mix, then layer in the kimchi, cabbage, carrots, onion, tofu, and cilantro, and then add the dry bundle of noodles on top.

Seal the jar then store in the refrigerator for up to 4 days.

When ready to eat, allow the jar to come to room temperature. Pour in 2 cups boiling water over the noodle jar ingredients, cover with a lid, and allow to sit for at least 3 minutes or until the noodles have completely softened.

So normally what I will do at the start of the week is prep some basics. I'll typically prep enough grains to last three days, cook or make sure I have some canned lentils on hand in the pantry, then make one to two sauces for the week. The sauces are key because after making them, I have enough to use for different meals during the week, and they help add so much flavor without me having to do extra work. And this concept works with lots of different sauces, which helps change things up and keep your meals feeling fresh and exciting.

Herby Cauliflower Stuffed Pita

SERVES 3 • PREP TIME: 15 MINUTES • COOKING TIME: 30 MINUTES

1 small head cauliflower, cut into 1-inch florets

1 tablespoon avocado oil, or more as needed

1 teaspoon garlic powder

½ teaspoon onion powder

½ teaspoon ground coriander

Kosher salt to taste

2 cups romaine lettuce, roughly chopped

1 15-ounce can (or 1 ½ cups cooked) small French lentils, drained and rinsed well

2 plum tomatoes, diced

2 to 3 tablespoons Pickled Red Onions (page 172) or 2 scallions, thinly sliced

¼ cup Zhoug (page 216), or more as needed

3 whole grain pitas

Roasted Garlic and Herb Tahini Dressing (page 211) or hummus (optional)

Preheat the oven to 425°F. Line a baking sheet with parchment paper.

Add the cauliflower to the prepared baking sheet, then drizzle with the oil and top with the garlic powder, onion powder, and coriander. Toss to evenly coat, using more oil if needed. Spread the florets out in a single layer cut side down, then generously season with some salt. Bake the cauliflower for 20 minutes on the bottom rack, flip, and then bake an additional 10 minutes until nicely charred around the edges and easy to pierce with a fork.

When cool enough to handle, roughly chop the cauliflower and place in a large mixing bowl along with the lettuce, lentils, tomatoes, and pickled onions. Add the Zhoug and a generous pinch of salt, then toss to evenly coat.

Warm a large sauté pan over medium-low heat and use it to warm the pita on both sides for a few seconds each until warmed through.

Cut the pita in half, spread the inside with a spoonful of tahini dressing if desired, then stuff with the cauliflower-lentil mix. Drizzle with more Zhoug, if desired, then serve and enjoy.

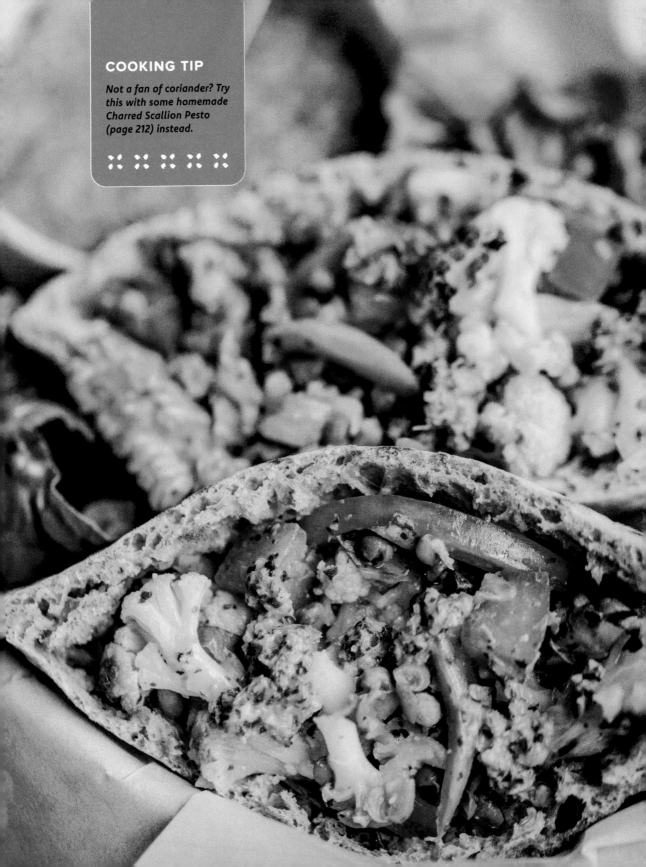

COOKING TIP

Not a fan of coriander? Try this with some homemade Charred Scallion Pesto (page 212) instead.

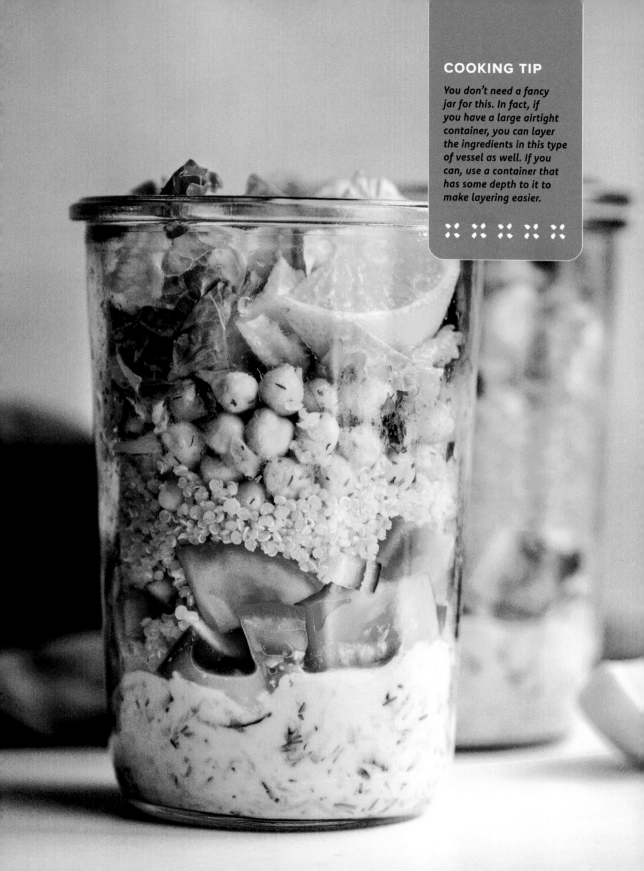

COOKING TIP

You don't need a fancy jar for this. In fact, if you have a large airtight container, you can layer the ingredients in this type of vessel as well. If you can, use a container that has some depth to it to make layering easier.

I always find lunch tricky. Often it inconveniently comes up when I'm in the middle of some-thing important. And if I have to stop what I'm doing to start making lunch from scratch or even just search for something, I'm more likely to just delay or skip lunch unintentionally. That's why I have made it a point to have something nice waiting for me in the fridge for lunch at all times. That way, there is no excuse, and I can just grab it and start eating right away. This recipe uses a simple tzatziki sauce as the base and is layered with veggies, marinated chickpeas, quinoa, and lettuce. A pretty meal with function because as you're layering, you can visually see the components of your meal, ensuring it is nutritionally complete. The way it's layered can also help with keeping your salad fresher for longer. All the delicate bits are at the top, which keeps them away from the wet elements that can turn them to mush. It works like a charm, and is, of course, super easy to assemble.

Chopped Veggie Tzatziki Jar

SERVES 3 • PREP TIME: 15 MINUTES • COOKING TIME: 20 MINUTES

FOR THE SALAD

1 cup quinoa, rinsed

2 cups vegetable broth

1 15-ounce can chickpeas, drained and rinsed

½ small red onion, minced

Zest and juice of ½ lemon

2 teaspoons red wine vinegar

1 garlic clove, grated or crushed with a garlic press

3 tablespoons fresh parsley leaves, minced

1 tablespoon minced fresh dill, stems removed

Kosher salt to taste

PREPARE THE SALAD

To a medium saucepan, add the quinoa and vegetable broth. Bring to a boil over medium-high heat, then reduce to a simmer and cover with a lid. Allow the quinoa to simmer for 15 minutes. Remove from the heat and allow to stand covered for 10 minutes, then fluff with a fork and al-low to cool.

While the quinoa cooks, marinate the chickpeas. To a medium bowl, add the chickpeas with the onion, lemon zest and juice, vinegar, garlic, parsley, dill, and a generous pinch of salt. Stir to combine and set aside to marinate in the fridge for at least 30 minutes.

Recipe continues

1 Persian cucumber, deseeded

½ cup plain unsweetened plant-based yogurt (choose one that is thick in consistency)

1 tablespoon extra-virgin olive oil

Juice of ½ lemon

1 garlic clove, grated or crushed with a garlic press

3 tablespoons minced fresh dill, stems removed

2 teaspoons red wine vinegar

FOR SERVING

3 Persian cucumbers, chopped

2 plum tomatoes or ½ cup cherry tomatoes, chopped

3 tablespoons kalamata olives, chopped

1 head romaine lettuce, chopped

3 lemon wedges

PREPARE THE TZATZIKI SAUCE

Grate the cucumber over a cutting board using a box grater. Once grated, scoop up the shreds in your hands and squeeze out any excess liquid into a bowl or sink to discard. Add the cucumber shreds to a small mixing bowl with the yogurt, oil, lemon juice, garlic, dill, vinegar, and a pinch of salt. Stir well to combine, then taste and adjust salt to preference.

TO SERVE

Divide the tzatziki evenly between 3 large mason jars or airtight containers. Then divide the cucumbers, tomatoes, and olives into the jars evenly. Add ½ cup cooked quinoa to each jar, then ½ cup of the marinated chickpeas, and top each jar with romaine lettuce and a wedge of lemon.

Seal the jars and place in the fridge for up to 3 days. When ready to serve, invert the jar over a bowl or plate, mix the salad together, and enjoy.

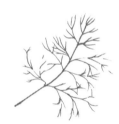

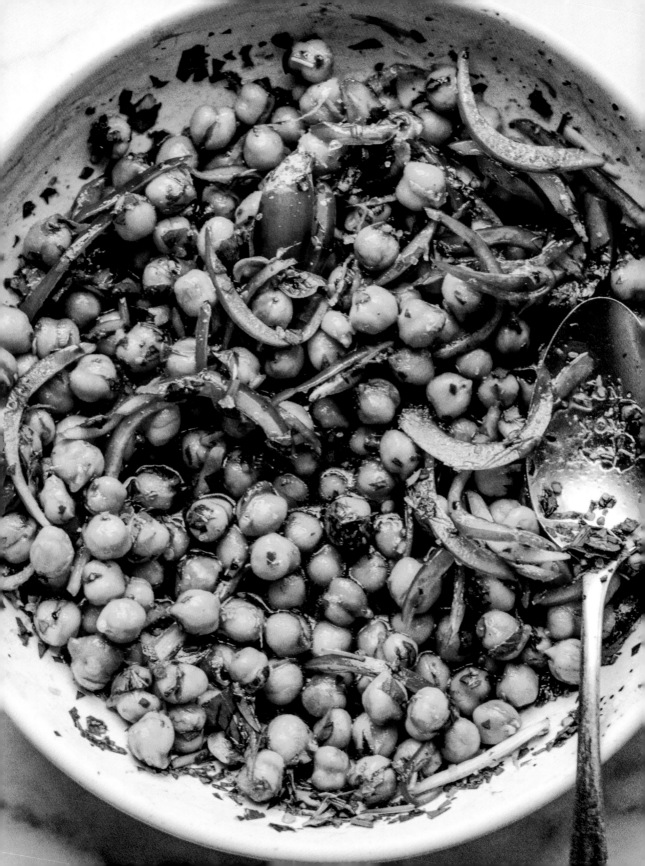

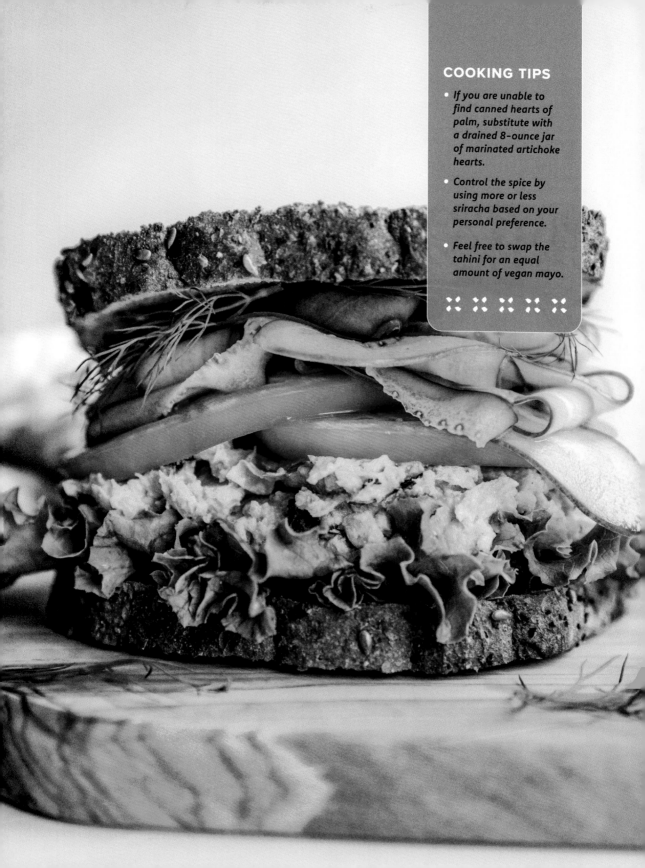

Oddly enough, one of my favorite things to eat when I was younger was tuna. Not the fancy stuff. Yep, the canned stuff, which many folks in the United States are accustomed to. It was a very common lunch item my mom would send me to school with. I'd eat it in a sandwich or with saltine crackers, and it would always hit the spot. Fast forward to now, when I'm looking for something similar, I turn to this chickpea version mashed together with hearts of palm to mimic the flaky texture of tuna. This, in combination with the nori, miso, and sriracha, gives it the right balance of umami and tang to satisfy my childhood nostalgia.

Spicy Tunaless Salad Sandwich

SERVES 3 • PREP TIME: 15 MINUTES

1 15-ounce can chickpeas or cannellini beans, drained and rinsed

1 cup canned hearts of palm

1 shallot, minced

1 celery stalk, finely diced

1 nori sheet

3 tablespoons good-quality tahini (see page 59)

2 tablespoons sweet relish

1 tablespoon Dijon mustard, plus more for serving

1 to 2 tablespoons sriracha

2 teaspoons yellow or white miso paste

Juice of ½ lemon

¼ teaspoon kosher salt

¼ teaspoon freshly ground black pepper

6 slices of whole grain bread

Lettuce

Tomato slices

Cucumber slices

To a medium mixing bowl, add the chickpeas and mash well with a fork. Place the hearts of palm on a flat cutting board, then mash and shred them with the same fork.

Add the mashed hearts of palm, shallot, and celery to the mixing bowl, then finely crumble the nori sheet overtop. If the nori is hard to crumble, blitz it in a mini food processor before adding to the bowl.

Next, add the tahini, relish, mustard, sriracha, miso paste, lemon juice, salt, and pepper, then fold everything together until evenly mixed. Cover and refrigerate for at least 30 minutes.

To assemble the sandwiches, spread some mustard between two slices of bread. Layer your sandwich with lettuce, then top with a few spoons of the chickpea mixture followed by tomato and cucumber slices, then enjoy.

You can use your layered jar salads to see if you are getting all the nutrients you need for a balanced meal. The goal should be to try and get half the jar loaded with some type of veggies, a quarter of the jar loaded with a protein, and the remaining quarter filled with an energizing starch. The rest can be accessorized to your preference to include things like healthy fats in dressings, nuts, and seeds. In this jar, the udon is our starch and sits in a delicious sesame dressing. We then fill half the jar with shredded veggies and top it with some tofu for protein. Super simple to assemble, and it makes for an easy grab-and-go meal that will properly fuel you through the afternoon.

Sweet Sesame Udon Noodle Jar

SERVES 1 • PREP TIME: 15 MINUTES • COOKING TIME: 3 MINUTES

FOR THE SWEET SESAME DRESSING

1 tablespoon good-quality tahini (see page 59) or vegan mayo

1 tablespoon reduced sodium soy sauce

1 tablespoon sweet chili sauce

Zest and juice of ½ a lime

2 teaspoons maple syrup

1 teaspoon toasted sesame oil

FOR THE NOODLE SALAD

1 serving instant, fresh, or frozen udon noodles

¼ cup shredded carrots

⅓ cup shredded cabbage

¼ cup sugar snap peas, cut on a bias

1 scallion, thinly sliced

3 ounces smoked tofu, Crispy Baked Tofu (page 114) or ½ cup edamame

2 tablespoons chopped fresh cilantro leaves

PREPARE THE SWEET SESAME DRESSING

In a small bowl, combine the tahini, soy sauce, chili sauce, lime zest and juice, maple syrup, sesame oil, and 1 tablespoon water. Whisk until smooth, then pour the dressing into a 16-ounce wide-mouth jar.

PREPARE MAKE THE NOODLE SALAD

Cook the noodles according to package instructions. Once cooked, rinse the noodles well under cold water to cool them down, then drain well and place into the jar with the dressing.

Layer on top of the noodles the carrots, cabbage, snap peas, and then scallions. Add your protein of choice, then top with the cilantro. Seal the jar and place in the fridge until ready to eat. Jars can be stored in the fridge for up to 3 days.

When ready to serve, give the jar a little shake, then dump it out into a large bowl. Stir the noodles and veggies into the dressing, then enjoy.

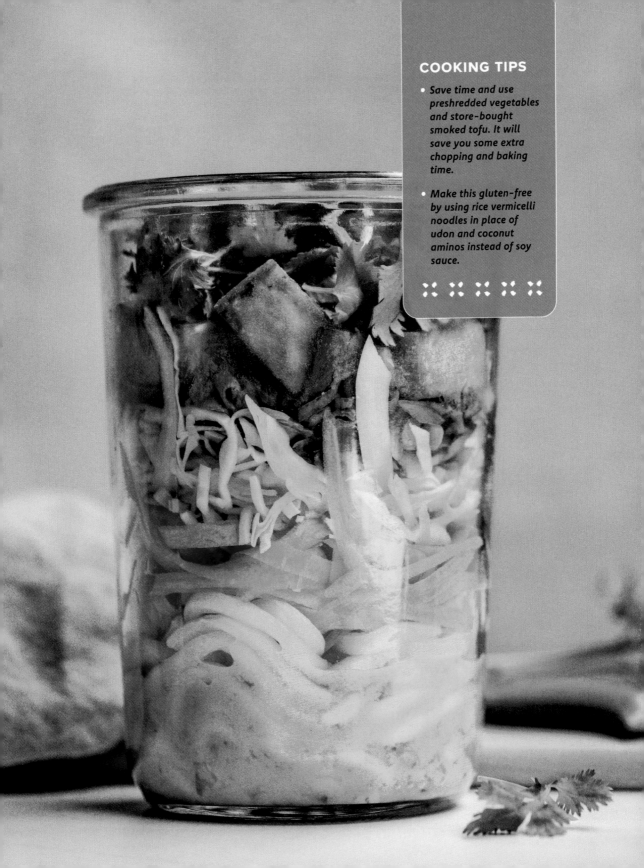

CHAPTER 4

Let's apply what we know about nutrition to build bowls that will help you GET THE NUTRIENTS you need. The soups, stews, pastas, and nourishing bowls in this chapter are all designed to mimic our PLANT PLATE METHOD so that they provide you with a good amount of PLANT-PROTEIN, steady energy to get you through the day, and lots of veggies. Use these as examples in the future to help you DESIGN YOUR OWN personalized nourishing bowl.

Nourishing Bowls

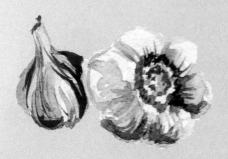

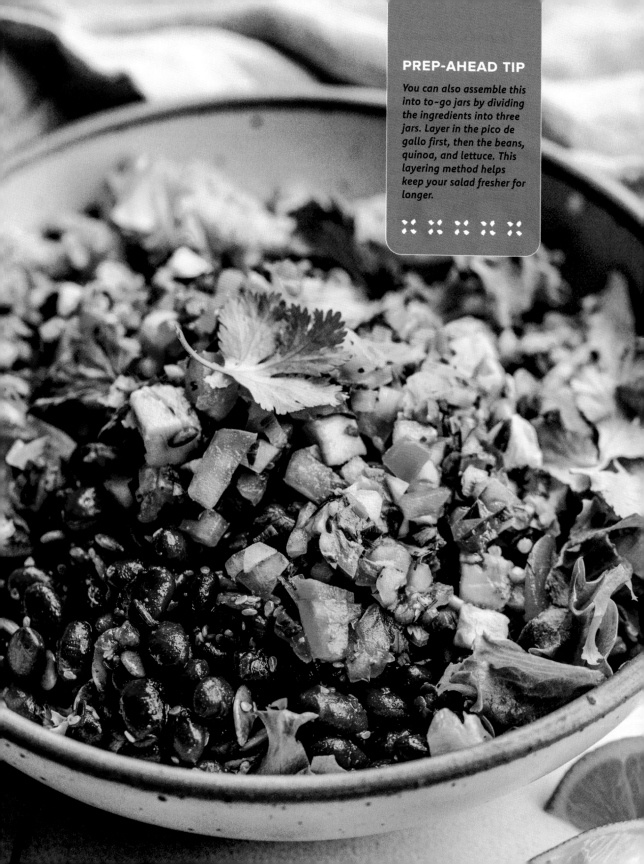

PREP-AHEAD TIP

You can also assemble this into to-go jars by dividing the ingredients into three jars. Layer in the pico de gallo first, then the beans, quinoa, and lettuce. This layering method helps keep your salad fresher for longer.

When I was working full time and going to night school, I didn't have much time for anything else. However, I had to make time for packing my lunch because I honestly couldn't afford not to. One meal I made frequently was something I called a "pico bowl." I would grab some store-bought pico de gallo (tragic I know, but convenient nonetheless!), frozen bagged quinoa, prechopped lettuce, and a can of black beans. I would heat up the quinoa, then put it in a lunchbox container with the beans and lettuce and top with a generous scoop of pico de gallo. This got me 3 very generous servings of food that actually tasted really good. This is a modified version of that meal that seasons the black beans to make it even more flavorful.

Pico de Gallo Bowl

SERVES 3 • PREP TIME: 15 MINUTES

1 15-ounce can black beans, drained and rinsed

1 garlic clove, grated

1 tablespoon reduced-sodium soy sauce or coconut aminos

2 teaspoons chili crisp oil

2 teaspoons maple syrup

2 teaspoons apple cider vinegar

½ teaspoon Tajín or chili-lime seasoning

¼ cup pepitas

1 tablespoon toasted sesame seeds

Kosher salt to taste

3 cups romaine lettuce, roughly chopped

2 cups cooked quinoa (see page 228)

1½ cups Avocado Pico de Gallo (page 206), or more to taste

To a large mixing bowl, add the beans, garlic, soy sauce, chili crisp oil, maple syrup, vinegar, chili-lime seasoning, pepitas, and sesame seeds. Toss together to combine, then taste and adjust salt to your liking.

To serve, divide the lettuce between three bowls, top with a third of the quinoa, beans, and pico de gallo.

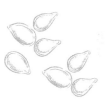

Fridays are noodle night in my home. It's seriously my favorite way to end a long workweek because it always feels like a tasty reward for all the hard work done. And while noodle night can vary week to week based on what we have on hand, I try to make it a point to whip up a batch of this creamy brothy soup as soon as the weather starts to cool down. The broth is protein-loaded thanks to a combination of peanut butter and soy milk, then it's topped with extra protein-rich tofu. It feels indulgent but finds a way to nourish and fill you at the end. A serious hug in a bowl that will help you recharge.

Creamy Miso Noodle Soup

SERVES 3 • PREP TIME: 15 MINUTES • COOKING TIME: 30 MINUTES

FOR THE TOFU

1 14-ounce block extra-firm tofu, pressed (see page xxxix) and cut into cubes

1 tablespoon tamari

1 tablespoon nutritional yeast

FOR THE SOUP BASE

2 tablespoons natural peanut butter or good-quality tahini (see page 59)

1 tablespoon maple syrup

1 tablespoon tamari

3 garlic cloves, crushed with a garlic press

1 tablespoon garlic chili sauce or sriracha

½-inch piece fresh ginger, grated or minced

1 vegan chicken vegetable bouillon cube or 1 teaspoon vegetable bouillon paste

2 teaspoons yellow or white miso paste

½ teaspoon ground coriander

¼ teaspoon ground turmeric

PREPARE THE TOFU

Preheat the oven to 425°F. Line a baking sheet with parchment paper.

Place the cubed tofu in an airtight container or resealable bag with the tamari and nutritional yeast, then toss to evenly coat. Place the tofu on the prepared baking sheet and bake in the oven for 25 minutes, flipping the tofu halfway.

PREPARE THE SOUP BASE

As the tofu bakes, to a blender cup add the peanut butter, maple syrup, tamari, garlic, chili sauce, ginger, bouillon cube, miso paste, coriander, turmeric, and 2½ cups water and blend until smooth.

Recipe continues

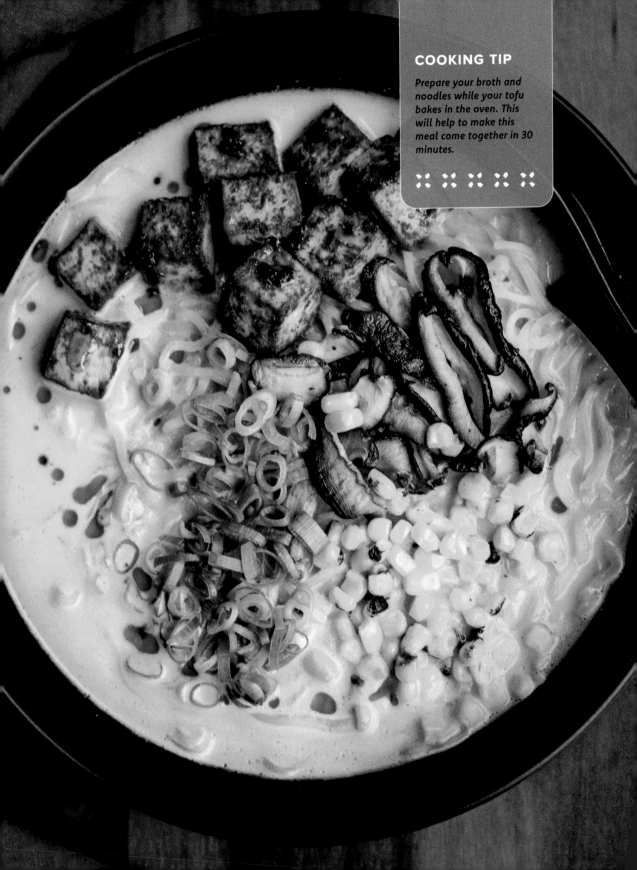

COOKING TIP

Prepare your broth and noodles while your tofu bakes in the oven. This will help to make this meal come together in 30 minutes.

4 ounces shiitake mushrooms, sliced

2 teaspoons sesame oil

Kosher salt to taste

2 scallions, thinly sliced

1 cup unsweetened soy milk

3 servings of wheat noodles or rice noodles

½ cup frozen corn, thawed

Chili oil for finishing (optional)

TO SERVE

Place a large saucepan over medium-low heat, and when hot add the mushrooms. Spread the mushrooms out on the bottom of the pan and allow to cook undisturbed for 2 to 3 minutes to release some water. Toss and sauté for an additional 1 to 2 minutes, then add 1 teaspoon sesame oil and a pinch of salt. Continue to sauté until well-coated, then transfer to a small bowl.

To the same pan, add the remaining 1 teaspoon sesame oil and the white ends of the sliced scallions. Sauté for 1 minute, then lower the heat, add the blended soup base, and let it simmer. Stir occasionally for about 2 to 3 minutes to allow the soup base to warm through. Once hot, pour in the soy milk and stir to combine. Remove the pot from heat.

Cook the noodles according to package instructions, then divide between the serving bowls. Divide and ladle the broth over the noodles, then top with the tofu, mushrooms, remaining scallions, and corn. Top with chili oil, if desired, then enjoy!

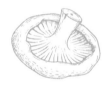

I think the thing that we don't appreciate enough when it comes to Indian cuisine, especially curries, is how nutrient dense it can be. Between the spices and the types of curries you can find, you can pack in an amazing amount of flavor and nutrients. And of the many types you can make, I prefer the ones loaded with lentils. Lentils are a rich source of protein and iron, and they require much less cooking time when making from scratch compared to other dry beans and chickpeas.

This is by no means the most traditional curry, but it uses all the spices I love to add for powerful flavor and heat. Since I make this often and try to mind saturated-fat intake, I do swap coconut milk for a little almond butter to add some fat and richness to this dish. Feel free to see the Cooking Tip for the coconut version. Lastly, if you have difficulty finding specific spices, I recommend that you visit your local Indian market where you'll find all the spices you need.

Go-To High-Protein Red Lentil Curry

SERVES 4 • PREP TIME: 15 MINUTES • COOKING TIME: 35 MINUTES

1 tablespoon avocado oil

1 bay leaf

1 teaspoon cumin seeds

2 shallots, diced

1 to 2 serrano peppers, diced (use less, deseed, or omit for less spice)

Kosher salt to taste

5 garlic cloves, crushed with a garlic press

1-inch piece fresh ginger, grated

3 plum tomatoes, diced

½ teaspoon garam masala

½ teaspoon Kashmiri chili pepper

½ teaspoon ground coriander

Heat the oil in a large skillet over medium-low heat. Once the oil is hot, add the bay leaf and cumin seeds and toast them for 45 seconds or until fragrant.

Add in the shallots and serrano peppers, along with a pinch of salt, and continue to sauté for 2 minutes until the shallots have softened.

Stir in the garlic and ginger and continue to cook and sauté until fragrant, about 1 minute.

Add in the tomatoes with another pinch of salt. Stir well to combine and cook the tomatoes until they start to break down, stirring frequently, about 5 minutes.

Next, add the garam masala, chili pepper, coriander, turmeric, and pepper, stirring them into the tomato mixture. Pour in the lentils and vegetable broth, then stir well. Raise the burner to medium heat and allow the lentils to come to a low boil.

Recipe continues

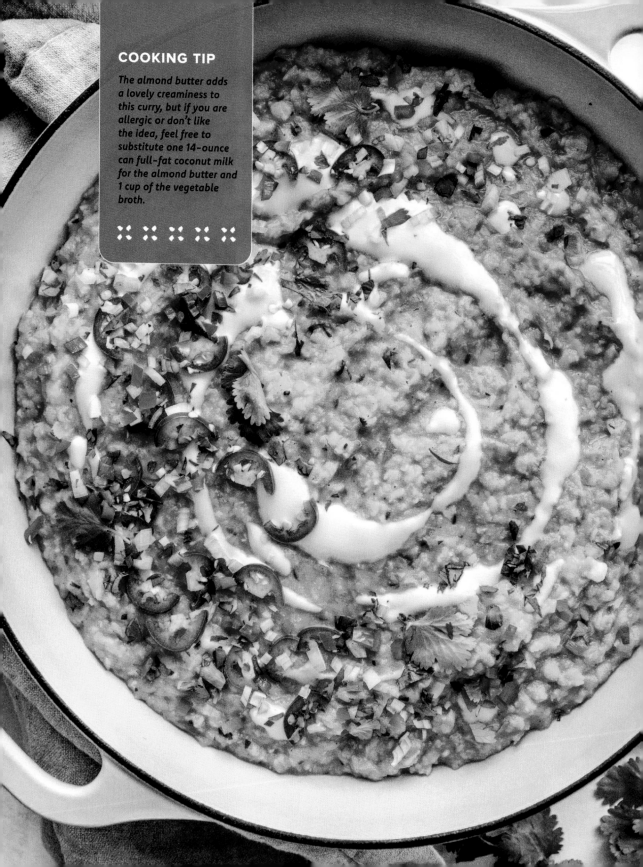

COOKING TIP

The almond butter adds a lovely creaminess to this curry, but if you are allergic or don't like the idea, feel free to substitute one 14-ounce can full-fat coconut milk for the almond butter and 1 cup of the vegetable broth.

¼ teaspoon ground turmeric

¼ teaspoon freshly ground black pepper

1 cup dried red lentils, rinsed

3 ½ cups vegetable broth

3 tablespoons natural almond butter or good-quality tahini (see page 59)

Juice of ½ lemon

Kosher salt to taste

Cooked rice (see page 228) or Sweet Potato Flatbread (page 167), for serving

Reduce the heat to a simmer and cover the pan with a lid and cook for 20 to 25 minutes or until the lentils have fully cooked through.

Remove the lid and stir in the almond butter until fully incorporated. Remove the pan from heat and add the lemon juice. Stir well, then taste and adjust salt to preference before serving.

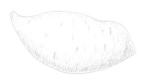

For me, every meal is made better with rice. It is one of the main reasons why rice bowls are a constant in my day-to-day eating. Not to mention, I feel that rice bowls give you an opportunity to see how you are balancing your plate. Loading your bowl with bright-colored veggies and including a plant-protein like tofu or legumes helps to make a meal feel more complete and satisfying. It also gives you a framework to modify and change your plate up to suit your own individual needs. And regardless of how that looks, you can still smother it in a delicious, sweet tahini-hoisin sauce to make it even better.

Sweet Hoisin–Glazed Tofu Bowls

SERVES 3 • PREP TIME: 15 MINUTES • COOKING TIME: 30 MINUTES

FOR THE TOFU AND BROCCOLI

1 16-ounce block extra-firm tofu, drained and pressed (see page xxxix)

1 tablespoon tamari

Zest and juice of ½ a lime

2 tablespoons nutritional yeast

1½ tablespoons avocado oil

2 cups broccoli florets

Kosher salt to taste

¼ cup Sweet Tahini Hoisin Sauce (page 209), plus more for serving

FOR SERVING

2½ cups cooked rice (see page 228)

3 Persian cucumbers, peeled into ribbons or chopped

PREPARE THE TOFU AND BROCCOLI

Preheat the oven to 425°F. Line two baking sheets with parchment paper.

Cut the tofu into equal bite-size cubes and place in a large airtight container, then top with the tamari, lime zest and juice, nutritional yeast, and 1 tablespoon of oil. Seal the container with a lid and give the container a few shakes to coat the tofu evenly.

Place the tofu on one of the prepared baking sheets with space between each piece, then place in the oven on the top rack to roast for 20 minutes. Flip the tofu and return to the oven for another 10 minutes or until golden.

On the second parchment-lined baking sheet, add the broccoli florets and the remaining ½ tablespoon of the oil with a pinch of salt. Toss the broccoli to coat and then spread the broccoli out on the tray, placing the broccoli cut side down. During the tofu's last 10 minutes of baking, place the broccoli in the oven on the bottom rack so it can roast for 8 to 10 minutes.

Transfer the tofu to a medium bowl, then pour the hoisin sauce over the tofu and toss to coat evenly.

TO SERVE

Divide the rice, cucumber, roasted broccoli, and tofu evenly between three bowls. Use additional hoisin sauce to drizzle over each bowl as desired and enjoy.

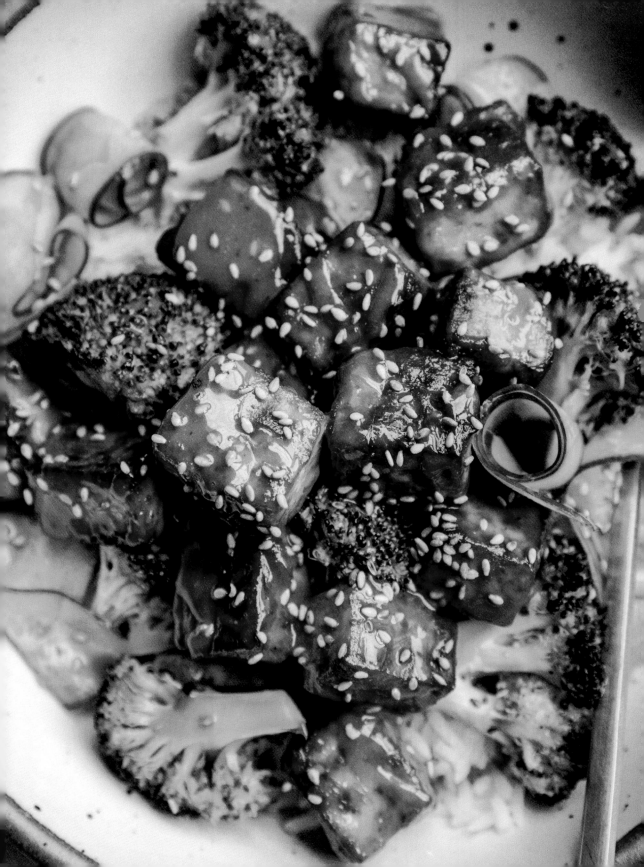

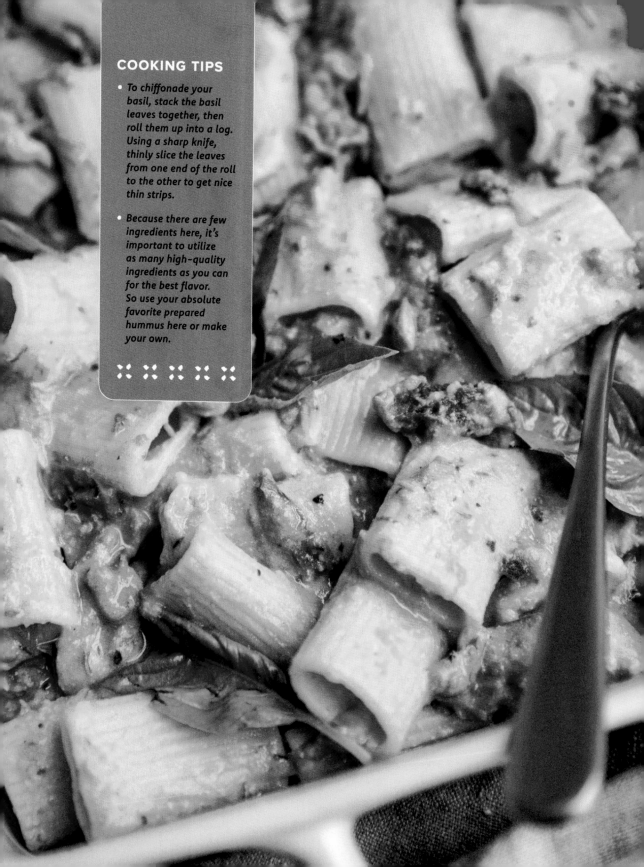

COOKING TIPS

- To chiffonade your basil, stack the basil leaves together, then roll them up into a log. Using a sharp knife, thinly slice the leaves from one end of the roll to the other to get nice thin strips.

- Because there are few ingredients here, it's important to utilize as many high-quality ingredients as you can for the best flavor. So use your absolute favorite prepared hummus here or make your own.

By now, a great majority of us have become familiar with or exposed to hummus in some way. *Hummus* is the Arabic word for *chickpea*, which makes sense as the main ingredient in this Middle Eastern spread is chickpeas. Once blended with tahini, lemon juice, garlic, and salt, you end up with a creamy dip that is traditionally served with pita or in sandwiches, salads, or grain bowls. And as food evolves and traditions are shared, new ideas come into play. So as out there as this concept might sound, hummus used as a base for pasta sauce is absolutely delicious. It adds a great deal of flavor, has the perfect creaminess, and is supercheap and easy to make.

Baked Hummus Pasta

SERVES 4 • PREP TIME: 10 MINUTES • COOKING TIME: 40 MINUTES

Kosher salt to taste

2 pints cherry tomatoes

4 garlic cloves

2 to 3 tablespoons extra-virgin olive oil

1 cup hummus

½ teaspoon dried basil

½ teaspoon dried oregano

½ teaspoon dried rosemary

8 ounces rigatoni

⅓ cup sun-dried tomatoes, julienned

3 tablespoons nutritional yeast

5 to 6 fresh basil leaves, chiffonade

Juice of ½ lemon

Freshly ground black pepper to taste

Preheat the oven to 400°F and bring a large pot of water generously seasoned with salt to a boil on the stovetop.

To an 8 × 12 × 2-inch baking dish, add the cherry tomatoes and garlic, drizzle with 1 tablespoon of oil, and toss to combine.

Make a well in the center of the baking dish and spoon in the hummus.

Top the hummus with the basil, oregano, and rosemary, and drizzle with the remaining 1 to 2 tablespoons oil, then place in the oven to bake for 30 to 40 minutes or until the tomatoes are blistered and juicy.

While the hummus bakes, prepare your pasta according to package instructions, cooking it until the pasta is al dente and reserving 1 cup of the pasta water before draining.

Once the tomatoes and hummus are done, carefully mash your tomatoes and garlic with a fork, then mix it with the hummus.

Add the reserved pasta water, sun-dried tomatoes, and nutritional yeast, and stir well to combine. Pour in the cooked pasta, thinly sliced basil, and lemon juice, then toss to coat in the sauce.

Adjust salt and pepper to taste, then serve immediately.

When you've had a long day at work, likely the last thing you want to do is spend a lot of time in the kitchen. On those nights, under thirty-minute meals are a must. Luckily, these noodles cook in just twenty minutes. I do take some short cuts to make this happen. I use steam-in-the-bag broccoli florets and thawed frozen edamame to help avoid extra pans and extra chopping. Toss it together with the flavorful noodles, and you have a whole balanced meal in a bowl.

20-Minute Cilantro Lime Noodles

SERVES 2 • PREP TIME: 5 MINUTES • COOKING TIME: 20 MINUTES

Kosher salt

2 tablespoons tamari

2 teaspoons packed light brown sugar

2 teaspoons yellow or white miso paste

Zest and juice of 1 lime

¼ teaspoon five-spice powder

¼ teaspoon red pepper flakes

¼ teaspoon white pepper

2 servings of your favorite wheat or rice noodles

2 tablespoons avocado oil

2 scallions, white and green parts thinly sliced

4 garlic cloves, thinly sliced

1½ cups edamame, thawed

⅓ cup fresh cilantro leaves, minced, plus more for serving

2 cups broccoli florets, steamed

1 tablespoon toasted sesame seeds or crushed pistachios, for serving

Bring a pot of water to a boil and add a generous pinch of salt.

Meanwhile, in a small bowl, combine the tamari, brown sugar, and miso paste. Using the back of a small spoon, lightly mash the mixture together until smooth. Add the lime zest and juice, five-spice powder, red pepper flakes, and white pepper, then whisk together until evenly mixed and set aside.

When the water is boiling, cook the noodles according to packet instructions. Drain well and set aside.

Heat the oil in a large skillet over medium heat. When hot, add the white parts of the scallions and sauté for about 1 minute to soften. Stir in the garlic and continue to cook until fragrant, about 1 minute.

Add the cooked noodles to the pan and stir them well into the scallion mixture. Lower the stovetop heat, then pour in the mixed sauce that was prepared earlier. Allow the sauce to simmer and thicken while stirring and evenly coating the noodles.

Add the edamame, cilantro, and broccoli and stir until evenly mixed together with the noodles. Serve and garnish with extra cilantro, green parts of the scallions, and sesame seeds.

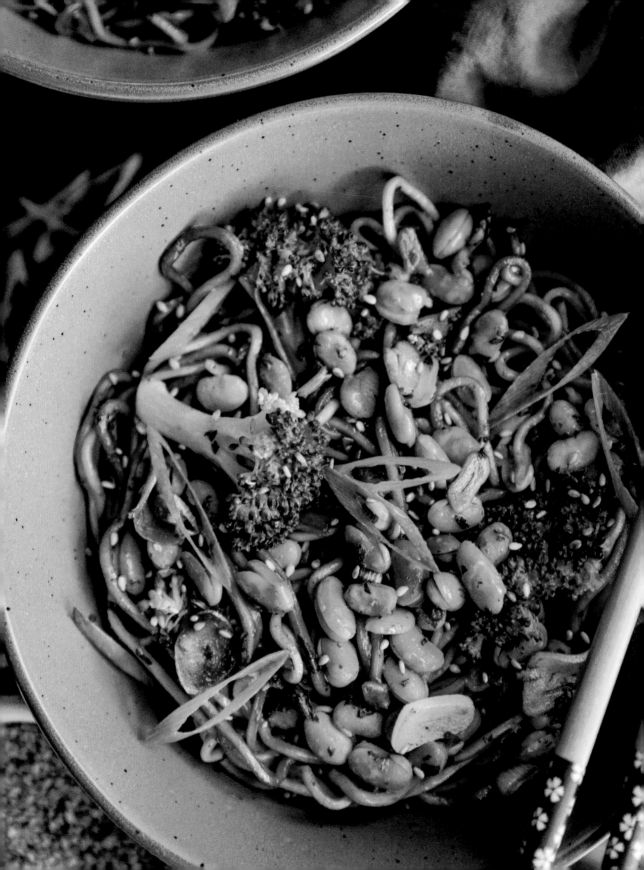

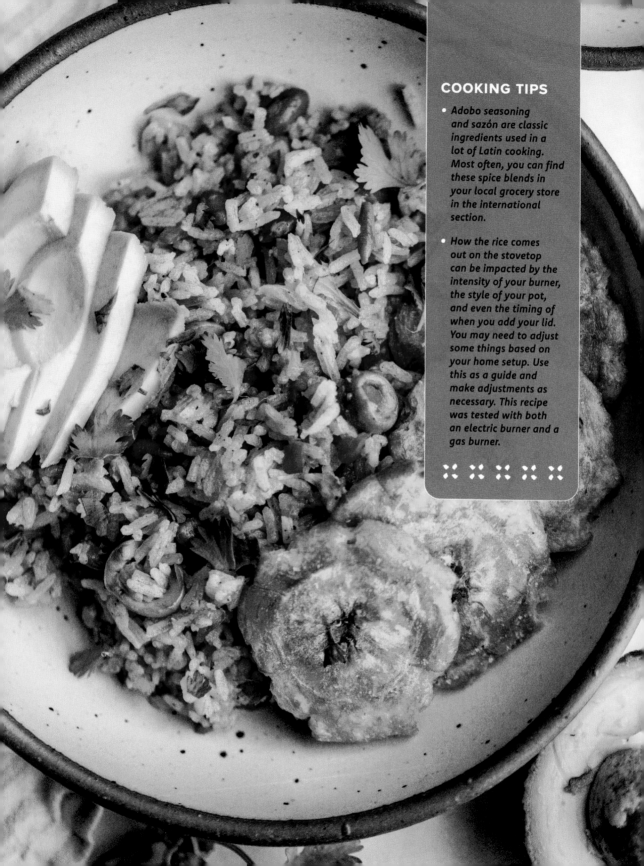

COOKING TIPS

- Adobo seasoning and sazón are classic ingredients used in a lot of Latin cooking. Most often, you can find these spice blends in your local grocery store in the international section.

- How the rice comes out on the stovetop can be impacted by the intensity of your burner, the style of your pot, and even the timing of when you add your lid. You may need to adjust some things based on your home setup. Use this as a guide and make adjustments as necessary. This recipe was tested with both an electric burner and a gas burner.

Moro is my favorite rice dish of all time and one of the most common dishes you'll see offered at a Dominican table. The best part, no matter how many Dominican homes you go to, is that every family has their own little tweak and addition that makes their Moro theirs. The smells and tastes all have their own stories, which I think is really beautiful. And when it's shared with family, you can feel the connection and love it provides. I think that's why whenever you ask a family member how they make their Moro, you'll get very vague responses. And good luck getting any measurements. So after watching my mother like a hawk over the years, I have learned to make my Moro this way. It is mine, I'm always happy to share, and I hope it can help you make your own special and tasty memories with your family.

Moro de Habichuelas

SERVES 6 TO 8 • PREP TIME: 15 MINUTES • COOKING TIME: 35 MINUTES

2 tablespoons avocado oil

½ medium white onion, finely diced

½ small green bell pepper, finely diced

½ small red bell pepper, finely diced

3 garlic cloves, crushed with a garlic press

1 8-ounce can tomato sauce

2 teaspoons adobo seasoning

½ teaspoon sazón

½ teaspoon freshly ground black pepper

1 vegetable bouillon cube or 1 teaspoon vegetable bouillon paste

¼ cup Spanish olives

1 15-ounce can no-sodium-added pinto beans or red kidney beans with liquid

¼ cup fresh cilantro with stems, roughly chopped with stems and leaves separated

3 cups white jasmine rice, rinsed

Kosher salt to taste

Heat a large heavy-bottomed pot with oil on the stovetop over medium heat. Once the oil is hot, add the onion and both bell peppers, then sauté until the onion becomes translucent, about 3 minutes.

Stir in the garlic and continue to cook until golden and fragrant, about 1 minute. At this point, pour in the tomato sauce, then sauté the mixture for 2 minutes before adding the adobo, sazón, and black pepper.

Continue to stir your tomato mixture for another 2 minutes, then add the bouillon cube, olives, beans with their liquid, and cilantro stems, then stir well to combine.

Pour in 2 ½ cups water and bring everything to a boil.

Once boiling, add the rice and stir well to evenly coat. Allow the rice to continue cooking, stirring regularly to remove any rice sticking to the bottom of the pot. When the rice has absorbed most of the liquid, stir the rice once more and add in the cilantro leaves. Lower the heat to the lowest setting and cover the pot with a tight-fitting lid to steam the rice for 25 minutes.

Remove the rice from the heat. Remove the cover and give the rice a stir. Cover the pot with the lid and allow to sit for 10 minutes. Fluff the rice again and season with salt to taste before serving. If after 25 minutes of steaming, your rice is hard and dry, place the pot back over the lowest heat setting with ¼ cup of water and cook covered for 5 additional minutes.

Beans carry great meaning for me. I've grown up eating them often thanks to my mom, so learning to make beans like hers has brought me great joy and peace. A lot of that has to do with how much comfort I associate with them. It was a way of communicating with my mom without really having to exchange words. I'd grab a bowl and if I was having a bad day, they instantly made me feel better. Or if I was feeling proud, it would feel like a big bowl of congratulations.

The first time I figured out how to make them, I took a bite and was brought back to the times my mom would sternly call us downstairs before the food got cold. Before we could even ladle any, she'd always ask, "Is it good?" Mom, it always is. And now, I can share these with you.

Habichuelas Guisadas

SERVES 6 TO 8 • PREP TIME: 15 MINUTES PLUS 8 HOUR SOAK TIME • COOKING TIME: 1 HOUR AND 20 MINUTES

1 pound dried beans (I prefer pink beans)

1 bay leaf

1 tablespoon extra-virgin olive oil

1 medium Spanish onion, roughly chopped

1 jalapeño, diced (optional)

Kosher salt to taste

1 tablespoon tomato paste

2 tablespoons store-bought sofrito or Dominican Sofrito (page 223)

1 cup kabocha squash or Yukon gold potatoes, cubed

1 teaspoon adobo seasoning

¼ cup packed fresh cilantro leaves

Cooked rice (see page 228), for serving

Avocado slices, for serving

In a large bowl, place the dried beans and cover them with water by 2 inches. Allow the beans to soak for 8 hours or overnight. You'll notice by then that the beans have doubled in size.

Drain and rinse your beans well, then place in a large pot with fresh water to cover them by 2 inches. Add a bay leaf and bring the pot to a low boil over medium-high heat. Continue cooking at a low boil, stirring occasionally for 1 hour until soft, then remove from the heat. (You can also use a pressure cooker to cook them in 25 minutes, allowing for 10 minutes natural pressure release.)

Place a second large pot over medium-low heat and add the oil. Once hot, add the onion, jalapeño (if using), and a pinch of salt and sauté until softened. Add the tomato paste and sofrito and continue sautéing for 2 to 3 minutes until fragrant.

Using a slotted spoon, scoop out the beans from the pot (reserving the liquid) and transfer them to the sofrito mixture. Add the squash, adobo, and cilantro, then pour in 4 cups of the bean liquid (fill in with water if needed). Stir to combine, then bring everything to a boil. Lower the heat to a simmer, then cover with a lid and cook for 15 to 20 minutes until the squash has softened.

Use the back of your spoon or a potato masher to lightly mash some of the squash and beans to thicken. If needed, add more salt to taste, then stir well and remove from the heat.

Serve with rice and avocado, and enjoy.

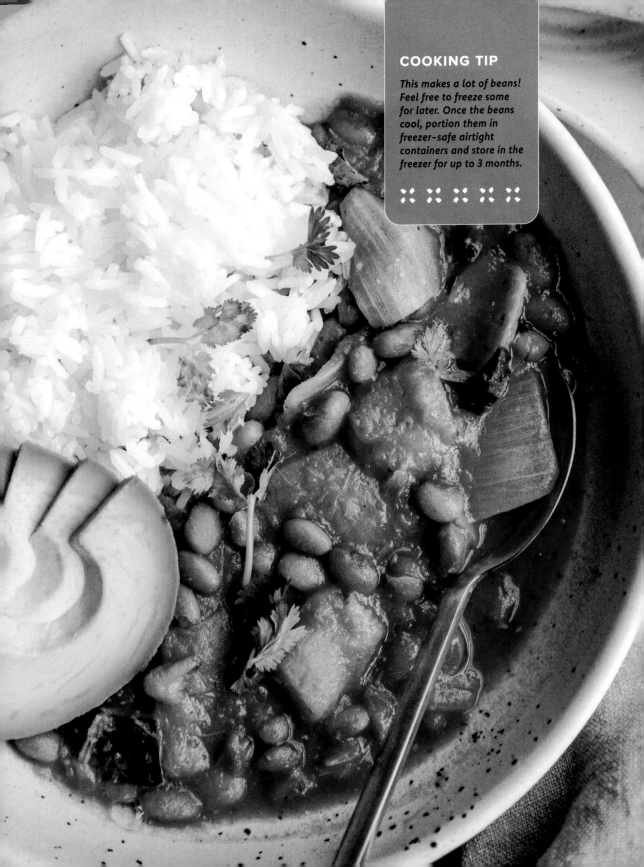

COOKING TIP

This makes a lot of beans! Feel free to freeze some for later. Once the beans cool, portion them in freezer-safe airtight containers and store in the freezer for up to 3 months.

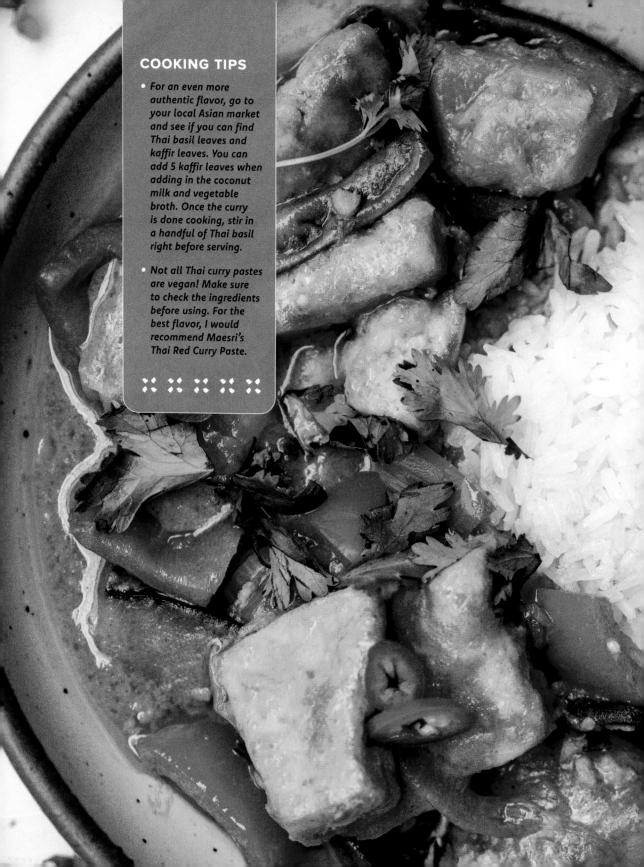

COOKING TIPS

- For an even more authentic flavor, go to your local Asian market and see if you can find Thai basil leaves and kaffir leaves. You can add 5 kaffir leaves when adding in the coconut milk and vegetable broth. Once the curry is done cooking, stir in a handful of Thai basil right before serving.

- Not all Thai curry pastes are vegan! Make sure to check the ingredients before using. For the best flavor, I would recommend Maesri's Thai Red Curry Paste.

I love eating out, but my wallet doesn't always feel the same. And honestly, if I can find most of the main ingredients to a dish I love and I can still make it in the time it would take to order and be delivered, I'm willing to do the work. There's also the added benefit that it gives you the power to adjust your food your way. You can add in more veggies, use a plant protein you love, or even adjust the level of spice to your liking. So when I'm craving a rich curry from my favorite restaurant, I tend to make this. I can find most of the ingredients in my small farm town, and if I get lucky, I might be able to find some extra ingredients to make it even more authentic (see Cooking Tips). The coconut milk really helps make this extra delicious, but feel free to sub in some oat milk if you happen to have an allergy or are minding your saturated-fat intake.

Thai Red Curry Tofu

SERVES 4 • PREP TIME: 15 MINUTES • COOKING TIME: 30 MINUTES

FOR THE BAKED TOFU

1 16-ounce block extra-firm tofu, drained and pressed (see page xxxix)

1 tablespoon tamari (see page xli)

2 tablespoons potato starch or 1 tablespoon cornstarch

1 tablespoon avocado oil

FOR THE CURRY BASE

1 14-ounce can full-fat coconut milk

2 shallots, sliced

3 garlic cloves, crushed with a garlic press

1-inch piece fresh ginger, grated

4 tablespoons Thai red curry paste

2 teaspoons fresh lemongrass, minced

1 teaspoon packed light brown sugar

PREPARE THE BAKED TOFU

Preheat the oven to 425°F. Line a baking sheet with parchment paper.

Tear the block of tofu into 1-inch chunks and place them in an airtight container or resealable bag. Add the tamari, potato starch, and oil, then seal the container and give the tofu a few gentle tosses to coat evenly.

Place the tofu on the prepared baking sheet and bake in the oven for 25 minutes or until golden in color.

PREPARE THE CURRY BASE

While the tofu bakes, heat a large skillet or wok over medium heat. Add 4 tablespoons of the coconut milk to heat through, then add the shallots, garlic, and ginger. Sauté for 1 minute until fragrant, then add the curry paste, lemongrass, and brown sugar. Continue to sauté for about 2 minutes.

Recipe continues

1 red bell pepper, chopped

½ cup fresh green beans, trimmed and cut into 2-inch pieces

1 cup kabocha squash or butternut squash, peeled and cut into 1-inch cubes

1 cup vegetable broth

Zest of 1 lime

Cooked rice (see page 228), for serving

Fresh cilantro, for serving

Lime wedges, for serving

Add the bell pepper, green beans, and squash, sautéing them into the curry paste to coat for about 1 minute. Pour in the vegetable broth and remaining coconut milk, then stir and bring to a simmer.

Allow the curry to cook for 5 to 8 minutes until the squash is fork-tender. Stir in the baked tofu and lime zest, then cook for 1 minute more. Remove from the heat and serve a portion of curry with some cooked rice, cilantro, and lime wedges.

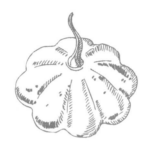

This one is all about timing, so if you time everything right, you can cook your whole dinner in just 30 minutes. The best part, the oven is doing most of the cooking for you. Just set up your trays with the chickpeas and your veggies, and while they roast in the oven, you can make a simple scallion rice salad to go with it. This whole meal is packed with bright zesty flavors that will make you want to keep making this on repeat.

Maple Dijon Roasted Carrots and Asparagus with Scallion Rice

SERVES 2 TO 3 • PREP TIME: 15 MINUTES • COOKING TIME: 30 MINUTES

FOR THE CARROTS AND ASPARAGUS

1 15-ounce can chickpeas, drained and rinsed

2 ½ tablespoons avocado oil

1 teaspoon garlic powder

1 teaspoon onion powder

Kosher salt to taste

1 ½ pounds carrots, roughly chopped into 1-inch pieces

½ teaspoon fennel seeds

8 asparagus spears, woody ends removed, cut on a bias

Freshly ground black pepper

PREPARE THE CARROTS AND ASPARAGUS

Preheat the oven to 425°F. Line two baking sheets with parchment paper.

Pat the chickpeas dry with a clean kitchen towel.

Place the chickpeas in a small bowl and add 1 tablespoon of oil, ½ teaspoon garlic powder and onion powder, and a pinch of salt over the chickpeas. Toss to evenly coat, then spread into a single layer on half of one of the prepared baking sheets.

To the same bowl, add the carrots. Add 1 tablespoon of oil and the remaining garlic powder and onion powder, then sprinkle the carrots with the fennel seeds and a pinch of salt. Toss to evenly coat, then spread into a single layer, making sure the carrots are cut side down, on the other half of the tray with the chickpeas.

Bake the carrots and chickpeas on the middle rack of the oven for 30 minutes, giving the chickpeas a toss after 15 minutes.

Place the asparagus on the other prepared baking sheet. Drizzle with ½ tablespoon of oil, then sprinkle with a pinch of salt and pepper and toss to coat. Place this tray in the oven on the bottom rack during the last 10 minutes of baking.

Recipe continues

3 cups cooked white rice

3 scallions, thinly sliced

2 teaspoons maple syrup

1 teaspoon Dijon mustard

1 garlic clove, grated

Zest of 1 lemon

Juice of ½ lemon

Kosher salt to taste

FOR SERVING

1 tablespoon maple syrup

1 teaspoon Dijon mustard

Maple Dijon Dressing
(page 205)

PREPARE THE SCALLION RICE

While everything bakes, place in a large mixing bowl the rice, scallions, maple syrup, mustard, garlic, lemon zest and juice, and a pinch of salt. Toss to evenly combine then set aside.

TO SERVE

Combine the chickpeas and all the vegetables together on to the same large baking sheet. Whisk together the remaining maple syrup and mustard then drizzle over top and toss to coat.

Serve the roasted chickpeas and vegetables over the scallion rice and top with the creamy Maple Dijon Dressing.

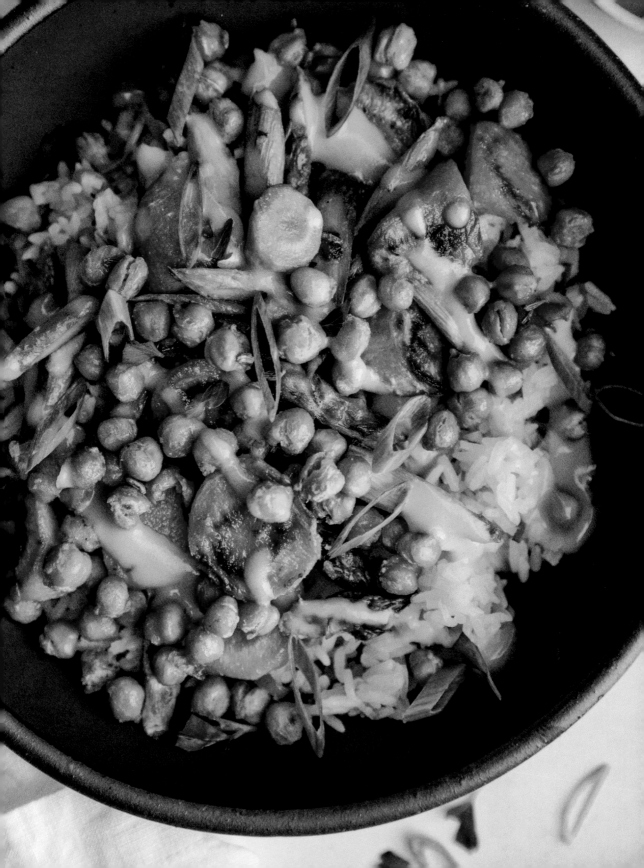

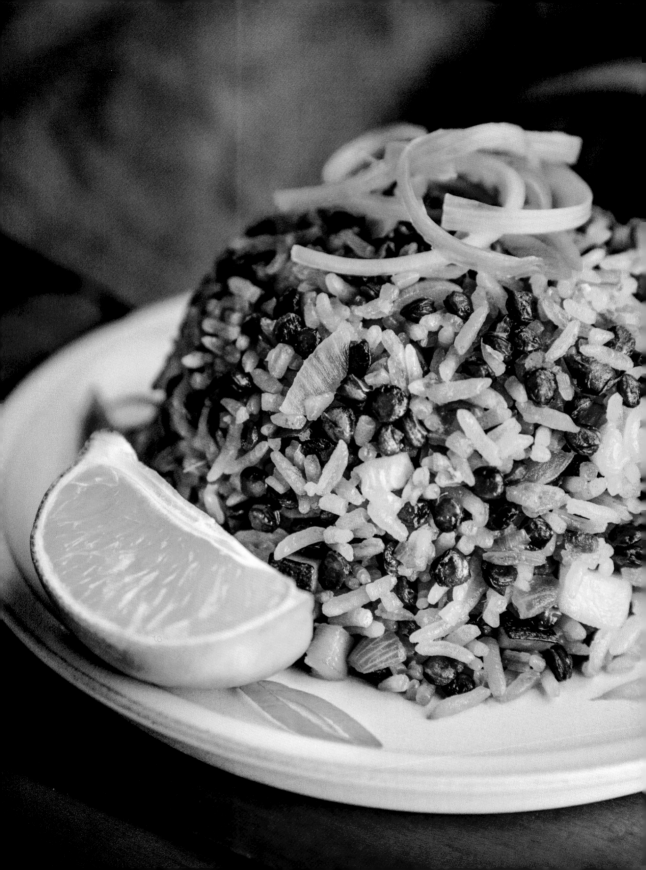

There are three very important principles you should know about fried rice. The first, have all your ingredients prepped before starting. Stir-frying anything goes by fast, and if you turn away for a second to chop something, things can burn and burn fast. And on the note of burning, high heat is a must. Keeping your pan nice and hot will give you the perfect even texture throughout your rice, so even if you don't have a wok, at the very least make sure your pan can withstand a higher temperature. Last, only use cold leftover rice. It's the rule! Cold rice is firmer and will not get mushy when stir-fried at a high heat. Plus, there's the added bonus of cooled rice developing resistant starches. As the name suggests, these starches resist digestion and function very similarly to fiber.

Scallion Ginger Lentil Fried Rice

SERVES 3 • PREP TIME: 15 MINUTES • COOKING TIME: 20 MINUTES

FOR THE CRISPY LENTILS

1 15-ounce can (or 1 1/2 cups cooked) small brown lentils or French lentils, drained and rinsed

1 teaspoon garlic powder

1/2 teaspoon onion powder

1 tablespoon avocado oil

FOR THE FRIED RICE

1 1/2 tablespoons tamari

1/2 tablespoon maple syrup

1/2 vegetable bouillon cube, crushed, or 1/2 teaspoon vegetable bouillon paste

1 teaspoon grated fresh ginger

1 to 2 tablespoons avocado oil

2 scallions, white and green parts thinly sliced

1/2 small yellow onion, diced

Kosher salt to taste

3 garlic cloves, crushed with a garlic press

1 medium zucchini, diced

3 cups leftover cold white jasmine rice

PREPARE THE CRISPY LENTILS

Preheat the oven to 425°F. Line a baking sheet with parchment paper.

If using canned lentils, drain and rinse them well, then place on a clean kitchen towel and pat dry. Add the lentils to the prepared baking sheet and top with the garlic powder, onion powder, and oil. Toss to evenly coat, then spread them out in a single layer on the baking sheet and place in the oven for 15 minutes, tossing halfway through.

PREPARE THE FRIED RICE

While the lentils roast, prepare your sauce. In a small bowl, combine the tamari, 1 tablespoon water, maple syrup, bouillon cube, and ginger and whisk together until the bouillon cube is mostly dissolved, then set aside.

Place a wok or a large skillet over medium-high heat. Add the oil, and once hot, add the white parts of the scallions and the onion along with a pinch of salt and sauté for 2 to 3 minutes until softened.

Add the garlic and zucchini and continue to sauté for an additional 2 to 3 minutes or until the zucchini starts to get golden around the edges.

Stir in the rice and start to break it up with your spatula and mix it into the vegetables. Pour in the prepared sauce and continue sautéing until the rice is evenly coated.

Add the roasted lentils and stir them into the rice, mixing until evenly distributed. Remove from the heat and serve, garnishing with the remaining green parts of the scallions as desired.

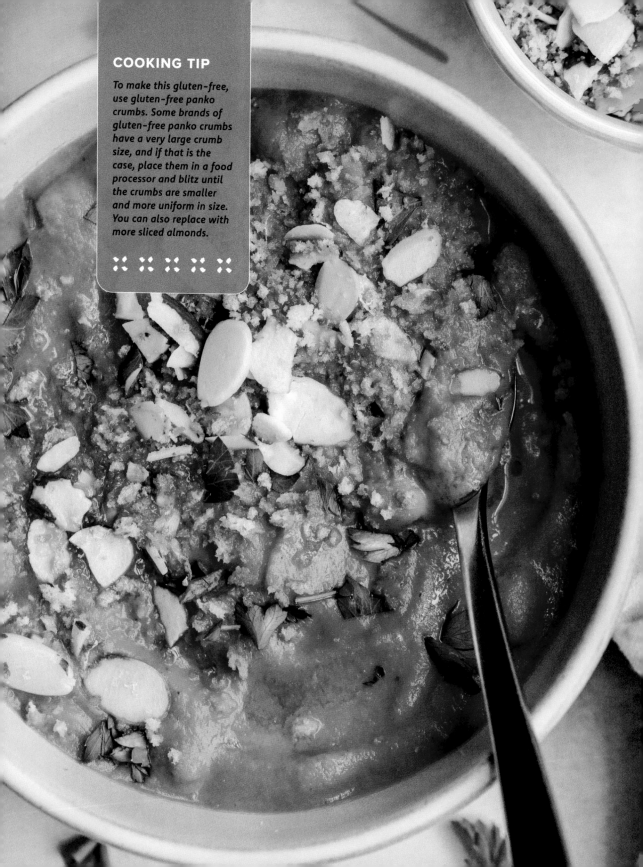

COOKING TIP

To make this gluten-free, use gluten-free panko crumbs. Some brands of gluten-free panko crumbs have a very large crumb size, and if that is the case, place them in a food processor and blitz until the crumbs are smaller and more uniform in size. You can also replace with more sliced almonds.

A giant bowl of creamy stewed tomatoes and bread is sometimes all anyone needs for a warm belly and soothed soul. Here we have protein in the form of beans and, instead of serving with a crusty slice of bread, topping with a crispy panko-almond crumb. A fully satisfying meal that can be cooked in less than 30 minutes!

Tomato Beans with Lemony Panko Crumbs

SERVES 4 TO 6 • PREP TIME: 10 MINUTES • COOKING TIME: 20 MINUTES

FOR THE PANKO CRUMBS

1 teaspoon extra-virgin olive oil

¼ cup panko crumbs or fine dried breadcrumbs

¼ cup sliced almonds

Zest of 1 lemon

Kosher salt to taste

FOR THE TOMATO BEANS

1 tablespoon extra-virgin olive oil

½ medium red onion, minced

1 red bell pepper, diced

Kosher salt to taste

4 garlic cloves, minced

2 pints cherry tomatoes, halved

¼ cup sun-dried tomatoes packed in oil, julienned

2 teaspoons smoked paprika

1 teaspoon Italian seasoning

1½ cups vegetable broth

2 15-ounce cans cannellini beans, drained and rinsed

Juice of ½ lemon

Handful fresh parsley, minced

PREPARE THE PANKO CRUMBS

To a large skillet over medium-low heat, add the oil. When the oil is hot, add the panko crumbs and almonds. Stir the mixture frequently until golden in color, about 2 to 3 minutes. Remove the pan from the heat and stir in the lemon zest and a pinch of salt, then transfer to a bowl and set aside.

PREPARE THE TOMATO BEANS

To the same skillet over medium-low heat, add the oil. Once the oil is hot, add the onion, bell pepper, and a generous pinch of salt. Sauté until the onion has softened. Stir in the garlic and continue to cook until the garlic is fragrant and golden, about 1 minute.

Add the cherry tomatoes and sauté until the tomatoes start to break down and become jammy, about 5 minutes.

Stir in the sun-dried tomatoes, smoked paprika, Italian seasoning, and vegetable broth. Once combined, use an immersion blender to blend the mixture until roughly smooth.

Fold in the beans, then reduce the heat to a low simmer and cover. Allow the mixture to simmer for 10 minutes. Stir in the lemon juice, then portion the creamy beans as desired and top with the toasted crumbs and a garnish of fresh parsley.

True comfort in a bowl—and this comfort doesn't need a lot of ingredients or that much time to achieve. For big flavor, we are relying on harissa paste. If you don't know, harissa is a hot chili pepper paste of North African origin with strong ties to Tunisia. While preparations for it vary household to household, this paste often uses a combination of peppers, spices, garlic paste, and oil. And while the condiment can be used as a dip or marinade, it also makes the perfect addition to stews. This stew would not be the traditional way to use this condiment, but it certainly packs in a lot of the rich flavor I'm looking for. It becomes even richer and more complex in flavor thanks to the addition of some peanut butter, which makes this stew extra creamy and velvety. Truly, the perfect bite.

Peanut Harissa Stew

SERVES 3 • PREP TIME: 10 MINUTES • COOKING TIME: 30 MINUTES

1 tablespoon extra-virgin olive oil

½ medium yellow onion, diced

Kosher salt to taste

5 garlic cloves, minced

2 to 3 tablespoons mild harissa paste

1 teaspoon smoked paprika

½ teaspoon dried thyme

½ teaspoon ground coriander

3 plum tomatoes, diced

1 medium sweet potato, peeled and diced

1 15-ounce can no-salt-added pinto beans with liquid

2 cups vegetable broth

3 tablespoons natural peanut butter

2 cups baby spinach

Cooked rice (see page 228), for serving

Crushed peanuts, for serving

Fresh cilantro, roughly chopped, for serving

Add the oil to a large saucepan, then place over medium-low heat. Once the oil is hot, add the onion along with a pinch of salt and sauté for 3 to 4 minutes until translucent. Stir in the garlic and sauté until fragrant, about 1 minute.

Add in the harissa paste, smoked paprika, thyme, and coriander and continue to sauté for 1 to 2 minutes.

Stir in the tomatoes with another pinch of salt and continue sautéing for 4 to 5 minutes until the tomatoes start to break down and fully soften.

Pour in the sweet potato, the can of pinto beans with liquid, and vegetable broth, then stir well to combine. Bring the mixture to a boil, then reduce the heat to a simmer. Cover the pan with a lid and cook for 15 minutes.

Add the peanut butter and stir until well combined, then cover and cook again for 5 minutes or until the sweet potato can be easily pierced with a fork.

Stir in the spinach, then remove the pan from the heat. Allow the spinach to fully wilt, then taste and adjust the salt as desired. Serve with some cooked rice and top with crushed peanuts and cilantro.

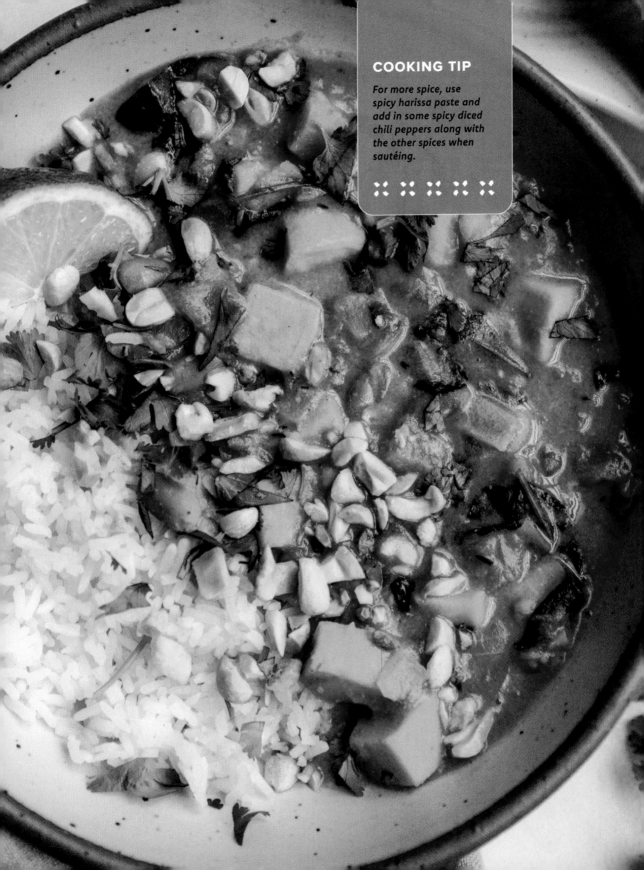

COOKING TIP

For more spice, use spicy harissa paste and add in some spicy diced chili peppers along with the other spices when sautéing.

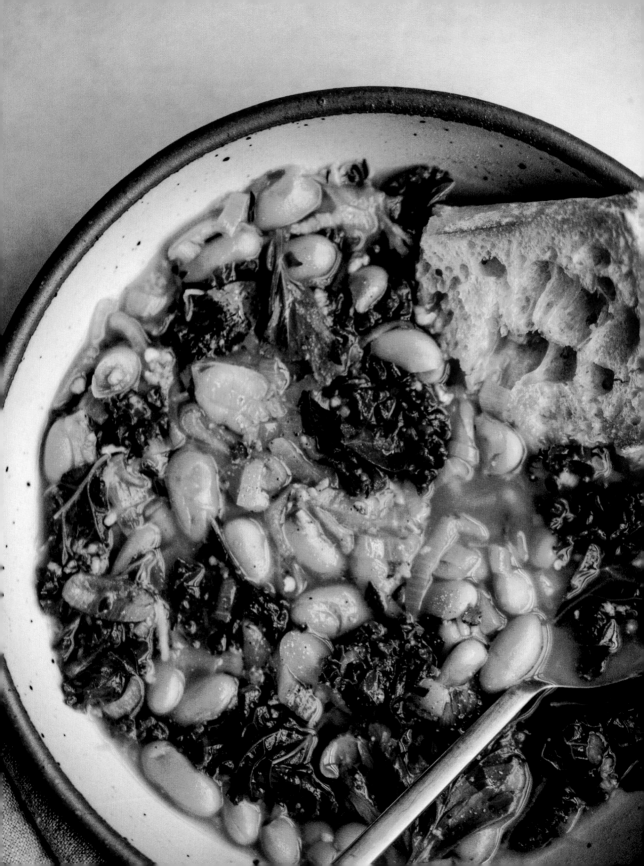

Okay, I get it. You don't have all the time in the world to cook fresh beans from scratch. And even if you have the time, maybe you forget to soak the beans or you don't have a fancy pressure cooker to help save the day. If you just have one pot and a few cans of beans, you can still make them incredibly tasty and, most important, fast. These brothy miso beans are for such circumstances and have come in handy when I'm in need of a nourishing speedy meal. The flavors don't disappoint either because we add some extra umami savory goodness into the broth to make up for it. Don't forget the crusty bread to help soak up every last bit of the broth.

Brothy Beans and Greens

SERVES 4 TO 6 • PREP TIME: 10 MINUTES • COOKING TIME: 20 MINUTES

2 tablespoons extra-virgin olive oil

2 shallots, sliced

1 tablespoon nutritional yeast

5 garlic cloves, crushed using a garlic press

1 teaspoon fresh thyme leaves

¼ teaspoon red pepper flakes (optional)

2 15-ounce cans cannellini beans, drained and rinsed

2½ cups vegetable broth

4 dried shiitake mushrooms

2 teaspoons yellow or white miso paste

1 cup kale, stems removed and roughly chopped

Juice of ½ lemon

Freshly ground black pepper to taste

Crusty bread, for serving

Add the oil to a Dutch oven or large pot and warm over medium heat. Once the oil is hot, add the shallots along with a pinch of salt and sauté until softened, 2 to 3 minutes.

Stir in the nutritional yeast, garlic, thyme, and red pepper flakes (if using) and continue to sauté until the garlic is fragrant, about 1 minute.

Pour in the beans, vegetable broth, and shiitake mushrooms, then stir well to combine. Bring the mixture to a simmer and cook for 8 to 10 minutes.

To a large cup, add the miso paste and ladle a small amount of the simmered broth over it. Whisk together until the miso paste dissolves, then add the mixture to the pot along with the kale. Stir until the kale turns a bright green and starts to wilt, then remove the pot from the heat.

Squeeze in the lemon juice and stir. Serve the beans warm with a few cracks of fresh black pepper and some warm crusty bread, then enjoy.

CHAPTER 5

When you eat a plant-based meal, you should FEEL SATISFIED. A big component to that satisfaction lies in not just FLAVOR but also making sure your meal is PACKED WITH PROTEIN. The following meals are designed to do just that.

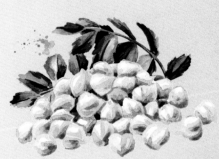

Nutrient-Packed Mains

This is my everyday tofu. The recipe has evolved more and more over the years, but it's generally the same and comes out perfectly every time I make it. The best part is, it's easy; you just coat it and pop it in the oven. No pan-frying necessary! And you can customize from here. Just use this as your base and add additional seasonings when needed. This tofu will help boost the protein in any meal you like.

Crispy Baked Tofu

SERVES 3 TO 4 • PREP TIME: 5 MINUTES • COOKING TIME: 40 MINUTES

1 block extra-firm tofu, drained, pressed (see page xxxix), and cubed into 1-inch pieces

1 tablespoon tamari

1 tablespoon apple cider vinegar or lemon juice

2 tablespoons cornstarch

1 tablespoon avocado oil

Preheat the oven to 425°F. Line a baking sheet with parchment paper.

To a large bowl, add the tofu. Pour the tamari and vinegar on top, then gently toss to coat.

Sprinkle the cornstarch on top, then drizzle with the oil. Gently mix until the tofu is evenly coated.

Transfer the coated tofu to the prepared baking sheet, allowing space between each piece.

Place the baking sheet in the oven on the top rack for 20 minutes, then flip the tofu. Bake for another 15 to 20 minutes until the tofu is crispy to your liking.

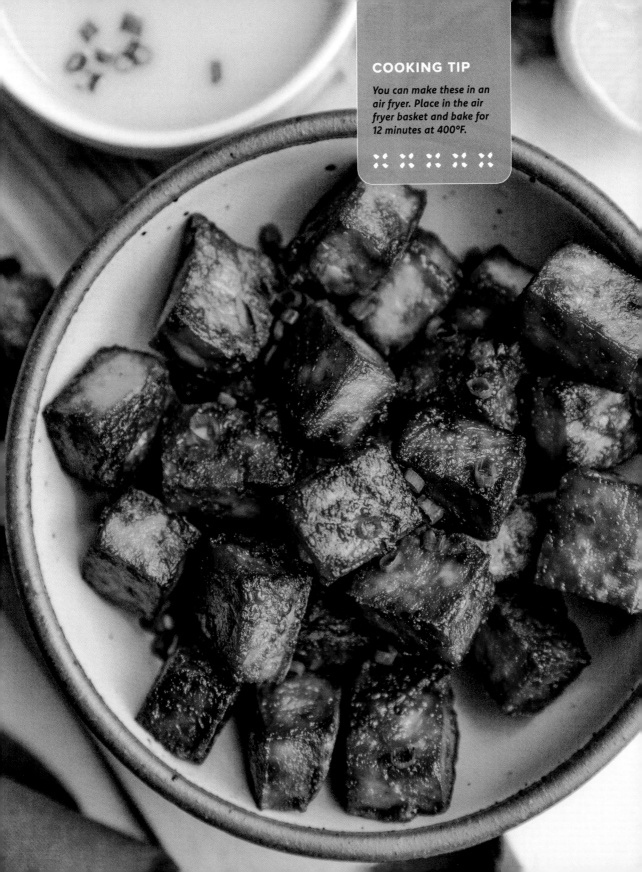

COOKING TIP

You can make these in an air fryer. Place in the air fryer basket and bake for 12 minutes at 400°F.

Once you understand the basics of tofu (see page xxxix), you can start flavoring it. I have four marinades you'll want to keep in your back pocket at all times, especially if you are a fan of prepping things in advance. These marinades will help infuse different flavors into your tofu and can be prepped in advance to make meal planning during the week unique, easy, and tasty.

Tofu Marinades Four Ways

Sticky Lemon Tofu Marinade

SERVES 4 • PREP TIME: 15 MINUTES • COOKING TIME: 25 MINUTES

Citrus in marinades not only helps flavor the outside of your tofu, but it also helps to tenderize and get more flavor into it. This marinade uses lemon as the star. Bake your tofu until it's tender, then thicken your marinade over the stove top to turn it into a tangy, sticky, sweet glaze to coat your tofu in.

4 tablespoons lemon juice

1 teaspoon lemon zest

1 tablespoon maple syrup

1 tablespoon red wine vinegar

1 teaspoon Dijon mustard

2 garlic cloves, crushed with a garlic press

¾ teaspoon kosher salt

½ dried thyme

½ teaspoon onion powder

1 16-ounce block extra-firm tofu, drained, pressed (see page xxxix), and cut into 1-inch pieces

Avocado oil spray or any high-heat oil

2 teaspoons cornstarch

Cooked asparagus (see page 161), for serving

Cooked quinoa (see page 228), for serving

To a small bowl, add the lemon juice, lemon zest, maple syrup, vinegar, mustard, garlic, salt, thyme, and onion powder, then whisk to combine.

Add the tofu to a large shallow container, then pour the marinade over the tofu and toss until completely coated. Seal the container and allow to marinate for at least 1 hour or preferably overnight.

When ready to cook, preheat the oven to 425°F. Line a baking sheet with parchment paper.

Remove the tofu from the marinade and place on the prepared baking sheet. Set marinade aside. Spray the tofu lightly with a little oil, then bake in the oven for 25 minutes, flipping halfway through.

Heat a large skillet over medium-low heat. To a small bowl, add the cornstarch and mix with 2 tablespoons water. Pour the reserved marinade into the skillet and bring to a simmer. Add the cornstarch slurry, and simmer until the sauce thickens. Add the baked tofu to the pan, then toss to coat in the sauce. Once the tofu is glazed, remove from the heat and serve with some cooked asparagus and quinoa.

Chili Miso Tofu Marinade

SERVES 4 • PREP TIME: 15 MINUTES • COOKING TIME: 25 MINUTES

Miso and chili oil help to infuse flavor into this tofu. You can then create a delicious savory, sticky sauce with the marinade that is leftover. If you want to avoid spice, just swap the chili oil with some sesame oil. This one I love to make when I'm in the mood for a quick takeout-like experience.

3 tablespoons low-sodium soy sauce

1 tablespoon chili oil

1 tablespoon maple syrup

1 tablespoon rice vinegar

2 teaspoons yellow or white miso paste

Zest and juice of 1 lime

2 garlic cloves, crushed with a garlic press

2 scallions, thinly sliced

2 teaspoons cornstarch

1 16-ounce block extra-firm tofu, drained, pressed (see page xxxix), and cut into 1-inch pieces

Cooked rice (see page 228), for serving

Steamed or sautéed frozen vegetables (see page 168), for serving

To a small bowl, add the soy sauce, chili oil, maple syrup, vinegar, miso paste, lime zest and juice, garlic, and scallions, then whisk to combine until the miso is fully dissolved.

Add the tofu to a large shallow container, then pour the marinade over the tofu and toss until completely coated. Seal the container and allow to marinate for at least 1 hour or preferably overnight.

When ready to cook, preheat the oven to 425°F. Line a baking sheet with parchment paper.

Remove the tofu from the marinade and place on the prepared baking sheet. Set the marinade aside. Bake the tofu in the oven for 20 minutes, flipping halfway through.

Heat a large skillet over medium-low heat. To a small bowl, add the cornstarch and mix with 2 tablespoons water. Pour the marinade into the skillet and bring to a simmer. Add the cornstarch slurry and simmer until the sauce thickens. Add the baked tofu to the pan, then toss to coat in the sauce. Once the tofu is glazed, remove from the heat and serve with some cooked rice and your favorite vegetables.

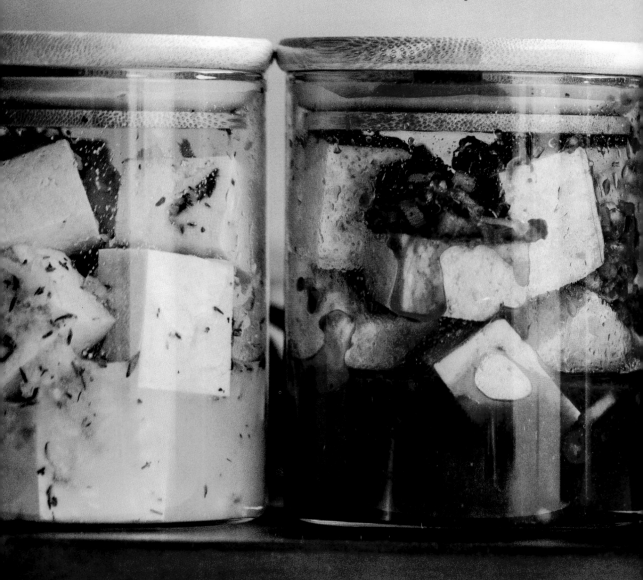

Sticky Lemon Tofu Marinade

Chili Miso Tofu Marinade

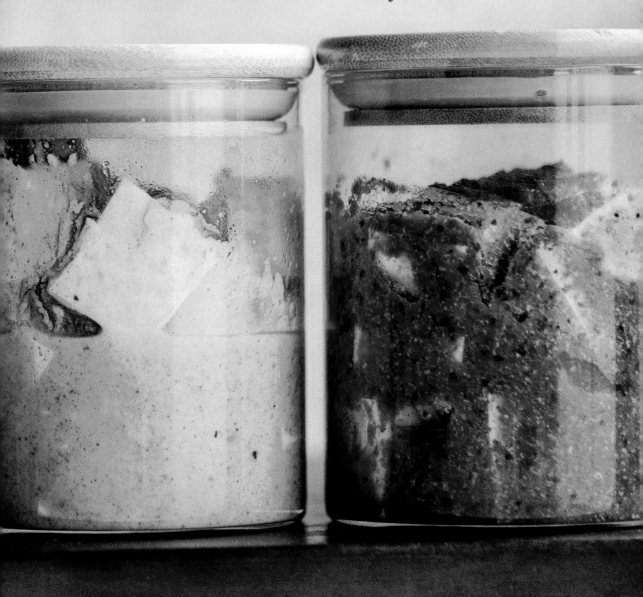
Tofu Tandoori

Tofu Guisado Marinade

Tofu Guisado Marinade

SERVES 4 • PREP TIME: 15 MINUTES • COOKING TIME: 45 MINUTES

Guisado is a lifestyle. If you aren't familiar with guisado, it refers to some kind of stewed meat. My mom would often make pollo guisado when I was growing up. I have since adapted the flavors she used in her stew to complement the plant-based proteins I eat today. This tofu guisado always hits the spot for me. I find it works the best when you marinate the tofu for a few hours, then cook it all down until it gets incredibly saucy and the tofu gets tender. Truly a taste of home for me.

4 tablespoons Dominican Sofrito (page 223)

2 tablespoons low-sodium soy sauce

2 garlic cloves, crushed with a garlic press

1 tablespoon tomato paste

1 tablespoon nutritional yeast

½ teaspoon adobo seasoning

½ teaspoon sazón seasoning

Juice of 1 lime

1 teaspoon light brown sugar

½ teaspoon kosher salt, plus more to taste

1 16-ounce block extra-firm tofu, drained, pressed (see page xxxix), and cut or torn into 1-inch pieces

Avocado oil spray or any high-heat oil

2 teaspoons extra-virgin olive oil

½ red onion, finely diced

1½ cups vegetable broth

Cooked rice (see page 228), for serving

Air-Fried Plantains (page 196), for serving

To a medium mixing bowl, add the sofrito, soy sauce, garlic, tomato paste, nutritional yeast, adobo, sazón, lime juice, brown sugar, and salt, then stir to combine.

Add the tofu to a large shallow container, then pour the marinade over the tofu and toss until completely coated. Seal the container and allow to marinate for at least 1 hour or preferably overnight.

When ready to cook, preheat the oven to 425°F. Line a baking sheet with parchment paper.

Remove the tofu from the marinade and place on the prepared baking sheet. Set the marinade aside. Spray the tofu with a little oil then bake in the oven for 20 minutes, flipping halfway through.

Heat a large skillet over medium-low heat with the oil. Once the oil has warmed through, add the onion with a pinch of salt and sauté for 2 to 3 minutes or until translucent.

Pour the marinade into the pan and sauté for 3 minutes. Pour in the vegetable broth and bring the mixture to a rapid simmer. Add the baked tofu to the pan, then toss to coat in the sauce. Lower the heat to a low simmer and cook for 20 minutes, stirring occasionally.

Remove from the heat and serve with some cooked rice and plantains.

Tofu Tandoori

SERVES 4 • PREP TIME: 15 MINUTES • COOKING TIME: 25 MINUTES

This marinade is inspired by classic tandoori chicken. Tandoori is typically marinated overnight in yogurt and spices, then grilled in a tandoor, a cylindrical clay oven. We are using tofu instead and using the marinade to help tenderize and flavor our tofu before finishing it off in the oven.

½ cup plain unsweetened plant-based yogurt

3 garlic cloves, crushed with a garlic pressed

½-inch piece fresh ginger, grated

½ teaspoon garam masala

½ teaspoon Kashmiri red chili powder

½ teaspoon ground coriander

¼ teaspoon ground turmeric

½ teaspoon kosher salt

Juice of 1 lemon

1 16-ounce block extra-firm tofu, drained, pressed (see page xxxix), and cut into 1-inch cubes

Avocado oil spray or any high-heat oil

To a small bowl, add the yogurt, garlic, ginger, garam masala, chili powder, coriander, turmeric, salt, and lemon juice, then whisk until smooth and uniform in color.

Add the tofu to a large shallow container, then pour the marinade over the tofu and toss until completely coated. Seal the container and allow to marinate for at least 1 hour or preferably overnight.

When ready to cook, preheat your oven to 425°F.

Soak a few 6-inch bamboo skewers in water for 15 minutes. Thread the tofu pieces onto the skewers and place on a bare baking sheet.

Spray or carefully brush the tofu with a little oil, then bake the tofu for 15 minutes, then flip and bake for an additional 5 minutes. Set the broiler on high and broil the tofu for 2 to 3 minutes until the edges get slightly charred, then enjoy.

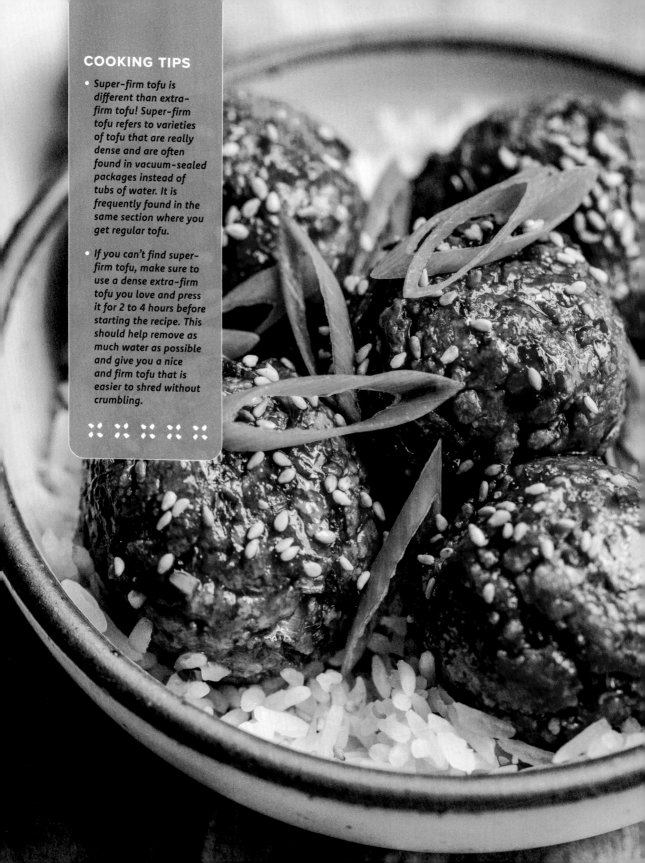

COOKING TIPS

- *Super-firm tofu is different than extra-firm tofu! Super-firm tofu refers to varieties of tofu that are really dense and are often found in vacuum-sealed packages instead of tubs of water. It is frequently found in the same section where you get regular tofu.*

- *If you can't find super-firm tofu, make sure to use a dense extra-firm tofu you love and press it for 2 to 4 hours before starting the recipe. This should help remove as much water as possible and give you a nice and firm tofu that is easier to shred without crumbling.*

Want to stick to healthy eating? Make it interesting! Sometimes that may include changing the way you might normally prepare your food. Take these tofu meatballs for example. Tofu is most often cubed before using in a dish. To change it up, try crumbling, seasoning, and shaping it into something fun like meatballs. This is especially great if a food like tofu on its own is something you aren't used to texture-wise. Learning new ways to enjoy foods like tofu helps open opportunities to add in more protein, iron, and calcium.

Sticky Ginger Tofu Meatballs

SERVES 4 • PREP TIME: 15 MINUTES • COOKING TIME: 40 MINUTES

FOR THE TOFU MEATBALLS

1 pound (454g) super-firm high-protein tofu (see page 122)

1 tablespoon soy sauce

1 tablespoon avocado oil or vegetable broth

½ cup all-purpose flour, spooned and leveled

⅓ cup panko crumbs or fine-dried breadcrumbs

1 teaspoon garlic powder

½ teaspoon onion powder

½ teaspoon ground ginger

½ teaspoon ground coriander

¼ teaspoon ground white pepper

½ teaspoon kosher salt

2 scallions, finely minced

PREPARE THE TOFU MEATBALLS

Preheat the oven to 400°F and line a baking sheet with parchment paper.

Crumble the tofu really well into a large bowl with your hands or a fork. Alternatively, you can also shred the tofu over the largest holes of a box grater. Make sure no large clumps of tofu remain, then add the soy sauce and oil and mix well to coat.

Add in the flour, panko, garlic powder, onion powder, ginger, coriander, pepper, salt, and scallions. Using your hands, knead the mixture together to evenly mix. When squeezed together firmly, the mixture should hold together. If your mixture is too dry, add 1 tablespoon of water, then mix and shape. If the mixture is too wet, add 1 to 2 tablespoons of panko until the mixture holds its shape.

Once fully combined, grab a 1½-tablespoon scoop of the mixture and shape it into a round ball. Place the tofu on the prepared baking sheet and repeat with the remaining mixture to form 15 to 16 balls.

Place the tray in the oven for 20 minutes, then flip the meatballs and bake for an additional 10 to 15 minutes until golden. Remove from the oven and allow to cool for 10 to 15 minutes to firm up further.

Recipe continues

1 tablespoon soy sauce

2 teaspoons grated
fresh ginger

1 garlic clove, grated

2 tablespoons maple syrup

1 teaspoon sesame oil

Zest and juice of 1 lime

2 teaspoons cornstarch

Cooked noodles or rice
(see page 228), for serving

Steamed vegetables or Easy
No-Mayo Slaw (page 157),
for serving

Toasted sesame seeds,
for serving

PREPARE THE SESAME GINGER GLAZE

While the tofu cools, to a small bowl, add the soy sauce, ginger, garlic, maple syrup, sesame oil, lime zest and juice, cornstarch, and 2 tablespoons water, then whisk well.

Place a large skillet or wok over medium heat. Once hot, add the sauce and allow it to come to a simmer, stirring occasionally.

Once the sauce starts to bubble, lower the heat to a simmer and add in the tofu meatballs. Toss to evenly coat in the sauce, then remove the pan from the heat.

Serve the meatballs over noodles or rice and with a side of veggies. Garnish with extra scallions and sesame seeds as desired and enjoy.

Have you ever shredded tofu? It's so simple and easy that I will find any excuse to shred it. Why am I such a fan? Shredding tofu creates more surface area, which helps to achieve the ideal flavor and also transforms the texture. So we're baking these shreds to crispy perfection and then flavoring with a delicious tinga sauce. The result, a completely different tofu experience than you've had before.

Tofu Tinga Tacos

SERVES 4 • PREP TIME: 15 MINUTES • COOKING TIME: 40 MINUTES

FOR THE TOFU

1 pound (454g) block super-firm high-protein tofu, drained and patted dry (see page 122)

1 tablespoon cornstarch

1 tablespoon soy sauce

1 tablespoon avocado oil

1 tablespoon adobo sauce from a can of chipotle peppers

FOR THE SAUCE

2 plum tomatoes

1 bell pepper, roughly chopped

½ yellow onion, roughly chopped

3 garlic cloves, peeled

2 chipotle peppers from a can in adobo sauce

½ teaspoon dried oregano

½ teaspoon dried thyme

½ teaspoon ground coriander

½ teaspoon vegetable bouillon paste or ½ vegetable bouillon cube, crushed

PREPARE THE TOFU

Preheat the oven to 425°F.

Place a box grater over a parchment-lined baking sheet. Grate the tofu over the largest holes on the grater to make shreds, then add the cornstarch, soy sauce, oil, and adobo sauce, then toss to coat. Spread out the mixture evenly on the baking sheet and bake in the oven for 15 minutes. Carefully toss and then bake again for another 5 to 10 minutes until golden.

PREPARE THE SAUCE

To a dry griddle or large heavy-bottomed pan over medium heat, add the tomatoes, bell pepper, onion, and garlic. The garlic only needs 1 minute on each side, so remove once cooked. Allow the remaining veggies to cook and sear on both sides for 3 to 5 minutes, flipping halfway through, until nicely charred on both sides.

In a blender, place the cooked vegetables, garlic, chipotle peppers, oregano, thyme, coriander, and bouillon paste and blend until completely smooth.

Recipe continues

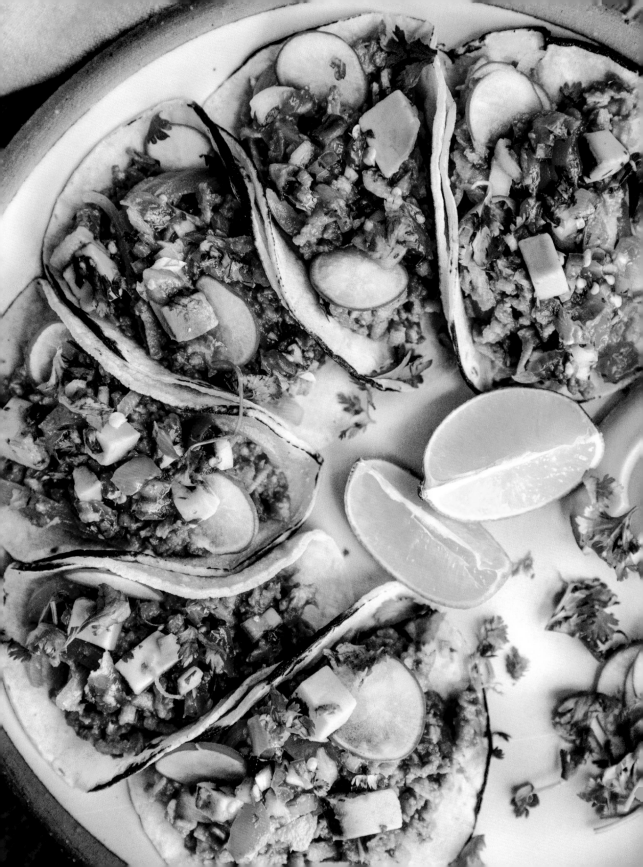

FOR COOKING

1 tablespoon avocado oil

½ yellow onion, thinly sliced

Kosher salt to taste

FOR SERVING

8 small corn tortillas

Avocado Pico de Gallo
(page 206)

Radishes, thinly sliced

TO COOK THE DISH

Heat a large sauté pan over medium-low heat, then add the oil to warm through. Add the onion with a pinch of salt and sauté until softened. Pour in the blended sauce and cook down to reduce the sauce in half, 7 to 8 minutes. Stir in the tofu and cook for 1 additional minute, then remove from the heat to serve.

TO SERVE

Heat up the tortillas for 30 seconds on each side in a medium sauté pan or over an open flame until softened, then serve with the tofu tinga and top with pico de gallo and radishes as desired.

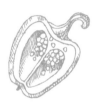

The only thing better than tacos is when the tacos are also incredibly budget friendly, too. And don't get me wrong, budget friendly does not mean you will lose flavor. These crispy buffalo tacos are anything but flavorless. They are bold, spicy, and made so much better by crisping them up in the oven. They also don't require a lot of ingredients. Just make the filling, stuff into your tortillas, and bake for a yummy, heart-healthy weeknight meal.

Crispy Buffalo White Bean Tacos

SERVES 4 • PREP TIME: 15 MINUTES • COOKING TIME: 30 MINUTES

2 tablespoons plus
2 teaspoons avocado oil

½ yellow onion, diced

2 garlic cloves, grated

1 teaspoon smoked paprika

½ teaspoon ground coriander

2 15-ounce cans cannellini beans, drained and rinsed

¼ cup buffalo sauce

3 tablespoons good-quality tahini (see page 59)

10 to 12 small corn tortillas

Jalapeño Lime Crema (page 219), for serving

Preheat the oven to 425°F. Evenly coat a bare sheet pan with 2 tablespoons of the oil and set aside to prepare the filling.

Heat a large skillet over medium-low heat with the remaining 2 teaspoons oil, then add the onion along with a pinch of salt and sauté until softened.

Stir in the garlic, paprika, and coriander and continue to sauté until fragrant.

Add the beans, buffalo sauce, and tahini and stir together to combine. With the back of your cooking spoon or a potato masher, lightly mash the beans. Continue to cook and stir until the mixture starts to bind together and thicken, then remove from the heat.

Soften the tortillas before adding the filling to prevent them from cracking. To do this, wrap 4 corn tortillas in a damp paper towel. Place them on a microwave-safe plate and microwave for 30 seconds. Take each tortilla and place on the greased baking sheet, giving a flip to coat both sides in oil. Spread 2 to 3 tablespoons of filling onto half of a tortilla and fold it over to close. To make sure your taco stays closed after folding, carefully flip the taco over so the filling placed on the bottom of the taco is weighing down the other side.

Arrange the folded tortillas on the greased baking sheet in a single layer with space between the tacos. Place in the oven to bake for 8 minutes, then carefully flip the tacos and bake for an additional 8 to 10 minutes until golden. Remove the baking sheet from the oven and allow to cool for 3 to 5 minutes to allow them to crisp up more, then enjoy.

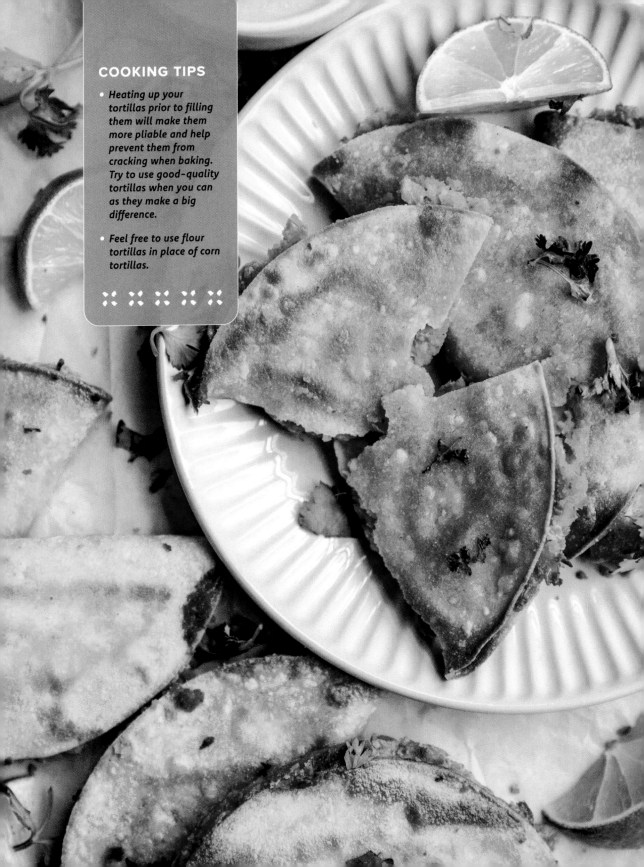

COOKING TIPS

- Heating up your tortillas prior to filling them will make them more pliable and help prevent them from cracking when baking. Try to use good-quality tortillas when you can as they make a big difference.

- Feel free to use flour tortillas in place of corn tortillas.

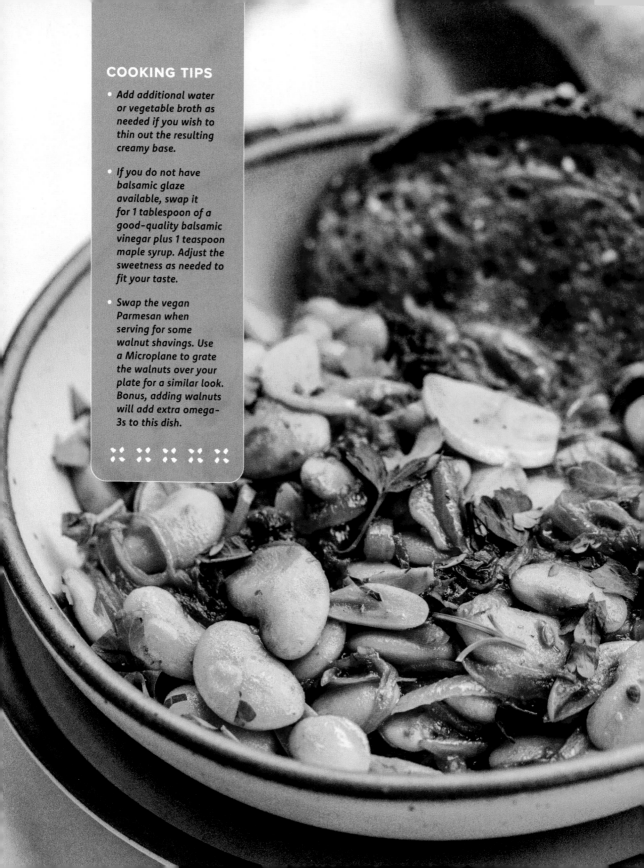

COOKING TIPS

- Add additional water or vegetable broth as needed if you wish to thin out the resulting creamy base.

- If you do not have balsamic glaze available, swap it for 1 tablespoon of a good-quality balsamic vinegar plus 1 teaspoon maple syrup. Adjust the sweetness as needed to fit your taste.

- Swap the vegan Parmesan when serving for some walnut shavings. Use a Microplane to grate the walnuts over your plate for a similar look. Bonus, adding walnuts will add extra omega-3s to this dish.

We're often taught that it's nutritious to eat the rainbow, but there is great value in the not-so-colorful dishes as well. Take these Caramelized Onion Butter Beans as a good example. This whole dish is beige minus the lovely garnishes I tend to always add to brighten the mood. And yet on its own, this dish can provide quite a number of useful nutrients. For example, the butter beans used in this dish provide up to 8 grams of fiber and offer a good number of vitamins and minerals like iron, manganese, and magnesium.

This nourishing meal also happens to use very few ingredients, making it a budget-friendly meal. To get the most flavor out of our base ingredient, onions, we are cooking them down until they are caramelized and jammy in consistency.

Caramelized Onion Butter Beans

SERVES 2 • PREP TIME: 5 MINUTES • COOKING TIME: 50 MINUTES

1½ tablespoons extra-virgin olive oil

1 large yellow onion, thinly sliced

Kosher salt to taste

4 garlic cloves, thinly sliced

¼ cup sun-dried tomatoes packed in oil, julienned

1 teaspoon dried oregano

½ teaspoon fennel seeds (optional)

¼ teaspoon red pepper flakes (optional)

1 tablespoon balsamic glaze

1 tablespoon nutritional yeast

1 15-ounce can butter beans, drained and rinsed

½ vegetable bouillon cube or vegan "beef" bouillon cube, or ½ teaspoon vegetable bouillon paste

Freshly ground black pepper to taste

Toasted sourdough bread, for serving

Vegan Parmesan cheese, grated, for serving

Heat a medium skillet over medium heat, then add the oil to warm through. Once the oil is hot, add the onion slices, give them a good stir in the oil, and spread them out evenly in the pan.

Allow the onions to cook, stirring occasionally, for 5 to 10 minutes or until you start noticing some brown streaks coating the bottom of the pan. Lower the heat to medium-low, add a pinch of salt and continue to cook for 20 minutes until the onions develop a deeper golden brown color, stirring every few minutes to make sure that the onions don't burn or stick too much to the pan. If the onions are sticking too much, add 1 to 2 tablespoons water to the pan as needed.

Add the garlic and sauté with the onions for 3 to 5 minutes or until they become fragrant and have softened.

Stir in the sun-dried tomatoes and oregano, as well as the fennel seeds and red pepper flakes (if using), and continue to sauté for about 2 minutes.

Add the balsamic glaze, nutritional yeast, butter beans, bouillon cube, and ¾ cup water, then stir well to combine.

Bring the mixture to a simmer and cook for 5 minutes. To thicken the broth, lightly mash a few butter beans with the back of your cooking spoon and stir everything to combine. Cook for an additional 5 minutes until your mixture is at your desired consistency. Serve a portion of the beans with some toasted bread, a pinch of black pepper, and vegan Parmesan cheese and enjoy.

I find that tempeh doesn't get the love and appreciation it truly deserves. And I think a lot of it comes down to preparation. This goes for just about everything you may want to eat, but learning how to properly utilize an ingredient makes a *huge* difference in how you enjoy it. For some, tempeh may come off as being bitter, and a lot of that has to do with the way it is normally made through fermentation, which gives it an earthy and mildly bitter flavor. However, you can balance the flavors of tempeh by following a couple of techniques that Indonesians use frequently with their traditional ingredient. First, pan-fry that tempeh and get it nice and golden. The high heat plus the oil can help mellow out some of the earthiness of your tempeh. Then, further balance it with some sweetness and some tanginess to truly bring out the best flavors. Once you get it flavored just right, you will then reap all the benefits of tempeh! It's high in protein and also contains iron, calcium, and fiber. So get on the tempeh hype train and make some!

Sweet Chili Peanut Tempeh

SERVES 3 • PREP TIME: 10 MINUTES • COOKING TIME: 20 MINUTES

2 tablespoons sweet chili sauce

1 tablespoon soy sauce

1 tablespoon mirin

Zest and juice of 1 lime

1 8-ounce block of tempeh

1 tablespoon plus 1 teaspoon avocado oil

1 shallot, thinly sliced

1 Fresno chile or jalapeño, thinly sliced (remove seeds for less spice)

2 garlic cloves, minced

1-inch piece fresh ginger, minced

¼ cup raw peanuts, roughly chopped

Kosher salt to taste

Cooked white rice or brown rice (see page 228), for serving

To a small bowl add the chili sauce, soy sauce, mirin, and lime zest and juice, then whisk together to combine before setting aside.

Cut the tempeh block in half, then cut each half-block crosswise into very thin slices. Keep the slices together to maintain the shape of the blocks, then cut the slices crosswise again to create little slivers.

Heat a large skillet over medium heat and add 1 tablespoon of the oil. Once the oil is hot, add the tempeh. Toss the tempeh in the oil, then spread it out into an even layer over the bottom of the pan.

Allow the tempeh to cook and sear undisturbed for 2 to 3 minutes or until it becomes lightly golden brown on the bottom. Lower the heat to medium-low, then give the tempeh a flip, spread it out again, and allow to cook undisturbed for 2 to 3 minutes. Repeat this process until the tempeh is a light golden-brown color all over.

Transfer the tempeh to a bowl and set aside, then add the remaining 1 teaspoon oil to the pan to warm through.

Once the oil is hot, add the shallot, pepper, garlic, ginger, peanuts, and a pinch of salt. Sauté the mixture in the oil for 2 to 3 minutes or until the onions have softened.

Add the tempeh back into the pan along with the sauce prepared earlier. Stir the tempeh into the sauce and continue to sauté until the tempeh is fully coated.

Remove from the heat and serve with some cooked white or brown rice.

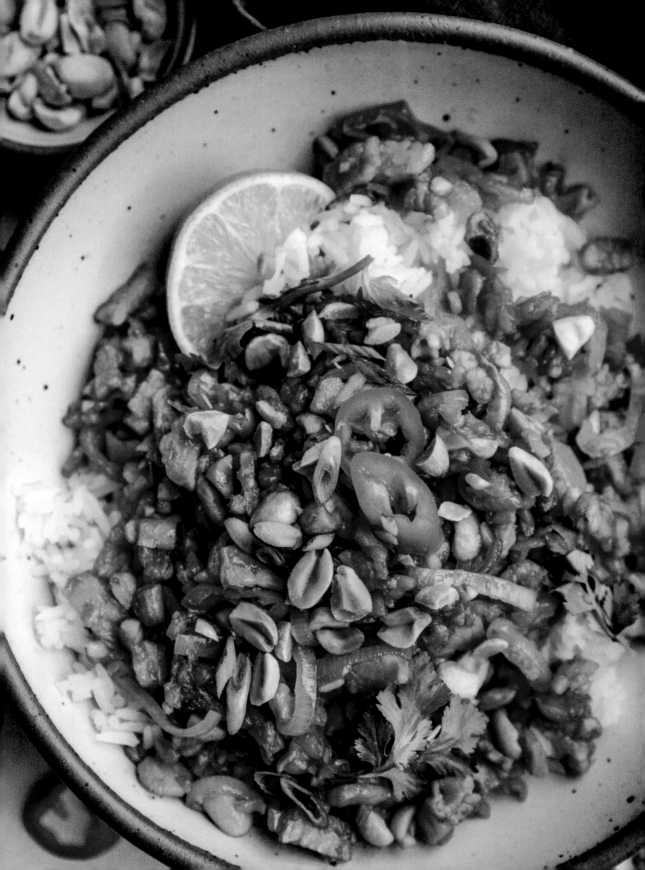

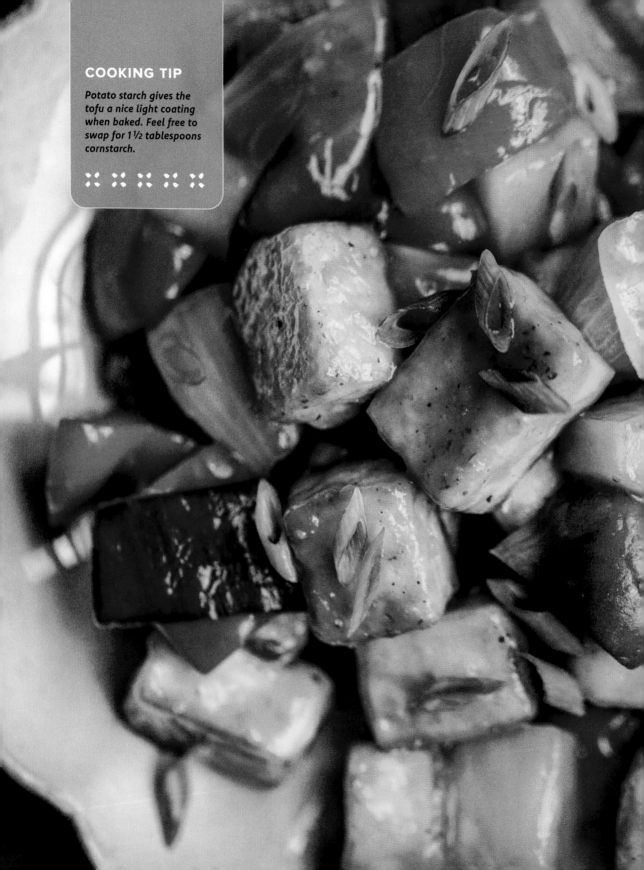

I'm not a dietitian who will tell you to never eat takeout. It's simply not a realistic expectation, and I feel that even things like taking a break from cooking can be worth splurging on now and then. However, if you are looking to save some money, making food at home isn't as challenging or expensive as you may think. Plus, depending on where you are, you might not have as extensive of a list of plant-based takeout options to choose from, so why not expand your menu at home? For me, I love this sweet and sour tofu dish I used to get from my favorite vegetarian Chinese restaurant in Philly. Since moving away, I treat myself by making this version. Once you prep all the ingredients, the cooking part goes by quickly. Glossy and perfect just like I remember.

Sweet and Sour Tofu

SERVES 3 • PREP TIME: 15 MINUTES • COOKING TIME: 40 MINUTES

FOR THE CRISPY TOFU

1 16-ounce block extra-firm tofu, pressed for 30 minutes (see page 122), drained, and cubed or torn into 1-inch pieces

1 tablespoon rice vinegar

½ tablespoon tamari (see page xli) or coconut aminos

2 tablespoons potato starch

¼ teaspoon white pepper

¼ teaspoon kosher salt

1 tablespoon avocado oil

FOR THE SWEET AND SOUR SAUCE

⅓ cup pineapple juice, from a can of pineapple in 100% juice

3 tablespoons maple syrup

3 tablespoons rice vinegar

2 tablespoons ketchup

1 tablespoon tamari or coconut aminos

1 teaspoon vegan Worcestershire sauce

1 tablespoon cornstarch

PREPARE THE CRISPY TOFU

Preheat the oven to 425°F. Line a baking sheet with parchment paper.

In an airtight container, place the tofu with the vinegar, tamari, potato starch, pepper, and salt. Shake well, then add the oil and shake again to coat.

Transfer the tofu to the prepared baking sheet, spreading it out evenly so there is space in between each piece. Bake in the oven for 20 minutes, flip, then bake again for 10 minutes.

PREPARE THE SWEET AND SOUR SAUCE

While the tofu bakes, combine in a small bowl the pineapple juice, maple syrup, vinegar, ketchup, tamari, Worcestershire sauce, and cornstarch. Whisk together to combine, then set aside.

Recipe continues

1 tablespoon avocado oil

1 garlic clove, grated or crushed with a garlic press

1 teaspoon grated fresh ginger

½ medium red onion, cut into 1-inch pieces

1 red bell pepper, cut into 1-inch pieces

½ green bell pepper, cut into 1-inch pieces

1 cup pineapple pieces, from a can of pineapple

Cooked rice (see page 228), for serving

STIR-FRY THE TOFU

Heat a large wok or skillet over medium-high heat with the oil. Once hot, add the garlic, ginger, and onion and sauté for 1 to 2 minutes until fragrant.

Add the red and green bell peppers and continue to sauté for 2 minutes. Add the baked tofu and pineapple pieces, then give the sauce a quick stir and pour it into the pan. Let it come to a rapid simmer and continue to cook and toss with the sauce for about 2 minutes to thicken.

Once the tofu and vegetables are coated and glossy, remove the pan from the heat and serve with some cooked rice.

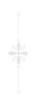

One thing that people tend not to understand when it comes to vegan or plant-based eaters choosing "meaty" protein alternatives is that texture can play a big part in the enjoyment of a meal. I think this is especially true for those who have grown up eating those meatier textures with meals. Honestly, it can feel like something is missing when those textures aren't present. Luckily, we live in an age when a lot of commercially prepared vegan meat options are available to help fill in this gap. You can also make relatively cheap alternatives at home, too, that are packed with protein. One of my favorites is seitan, which can give you 20 grams of protein per serving. I was always intimidated by it because most recipes I saw were a bit too involved and usually left me with a mushy and flavorless blob. Over the years, I've found a preferred method of preparing it that gives you a firmer and tastier option. This variation grills it in a pan and then coats it in a sweet, sticky sauce that will seriously satisfy.

Grilled Lemongrass Seitan Skewers

SERVES 4 • PREP TIME: 20 MINUTES • COOKING TIME: 15 MINUTES

FOR THE GLAZE

2 tablespoons maple syrup

1 tablespoon avocado oil

1 tablespoon tamari or soy sauce

1 lemongrass stalk, peeled and minced

1 small shallot, minced

1 garlic clove, crushed with a garlic press

FOR THE SKEWERS

1 cup vital wheat gluten

2 tablespoons nutritional yeast

1 teaspoon garlic powder

1 teaspoon ground coriander

½ teaspoon dried thyme

½ teaspoon onion powder

¼ teaspoon allspice

¾ cup vegetable broth

Soak some wooden skewers in water for at least 15 minutes to prevent your skewers from burning.

PREPARE THE GLAZE

To a small bowl, add the maple syrup, oil, tamari, lemongrass, shallot, and garlic and whisk together to combine, then set aside.

PREPARE THE SKEWERS

To a medium mixing bowl add the vital wheat gluten, nutritional yeast, garlic powder, coriander, thyme, onion powder, and allspice, then whisk together to combine.

To a large measuring cup or small bowl add the vegetable broth, almond butter, and tamari. Whisk together until nice and smooth, then pour the liquid mixture into the dry ingredients.

Using a rubber spatula, fold the ingredients together. As it starts to form a dough ball, use your hands to knead the remaining ingredients together until the dough ball is smooth and soft in consistency. Cover the bowl with a towel and allow to rest for 10 minutes.

Turn the dough ball out onto a smooth cutting board and divide the dough into 4 equal pieces.

Roll each piece into a short rope, then cut each rope into 6 short pieces, then thread the pieces onto the soaked wooden skewers.

Recipe continues

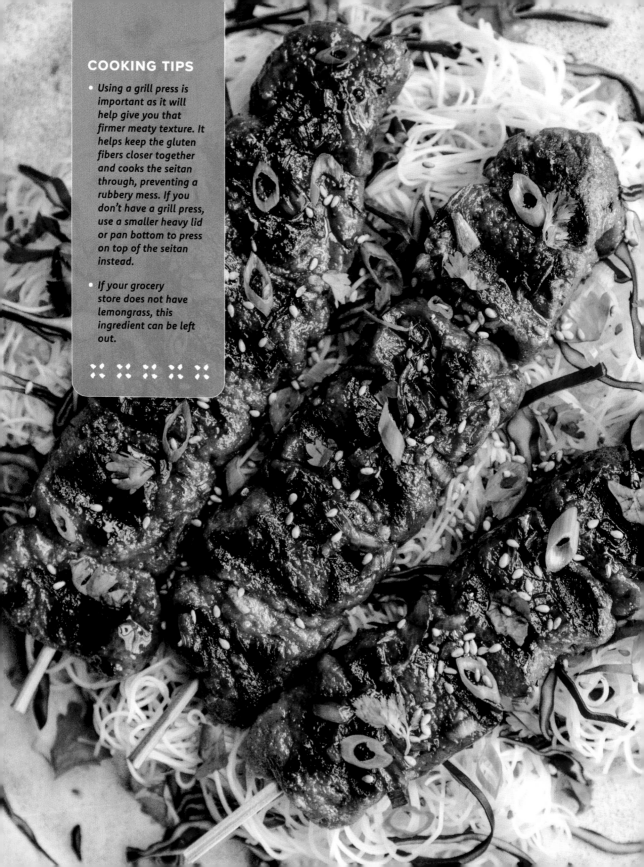

COOKING TIPS

- Using a grill press is important as it will help give you that firmer meaty texture. It helps keep the gluten fibers closer together and cooks the seitan through, preventing a rubbery mess. If you don't have a grill press, use a smaller heavy lid or pan bottom to press on top of the seitan instead.

- If your grocery store does not have lemongrass, this ingredient can be left out.

2 tablespoons natural almond
butter or tahini

1 tablespoon tamari

Avocado oil

Cooked rice (see page 228)
or rice noodles

Shredded carrots

Sliced cucumbers

Heat up a large nonstick grill pan brushed with oil over medium heat. Once the pan is hot, place the skewers on the grill pan and allow to cook undisturbed for 4 to 5 minutes or until some noticeable grill marks start to appear on the bottom.

Flip the skewers and place a grill press on top of them, then cook for an additional 4 to 5 minutes. Flip the skewers again, place the press over top and cook for an additional 2 to 3 minutes, then repeat on the opposite side. Once cooked, remove the skewers from the heat.

Heat a separate non-stick sauté pan over medium low heat. Pour in the sauce and allow it to come to a low simmer. Add the skewers to the sauce and rotate frequently as the sauce reduces and thickens. Once the seitan is evenly coated in the sauce, remove from heat.

TO SERVE

Remove the seitan from the skewers and enjoy with cooked rice or rice noodles and vegetables.

I adore falafel, and it was a go-to item I would order all the time when I first went vegan. It was an easy option available in a lot of spots that didn't require a ton of modifications to enjoy. It was also incredibly delicious. After eating it so often at restaurants or from street-food vendors, I wanted to learn how to make it myself. For traditional falafel, you use dried chickpeas that you soak in water, typically overnight. This process involves a long soak time, and I would often forget to do this before going to bed. So I started making a version that uses red lentils instead. They soak for significantly less time, and using the lentils provides a lot of protein in comparison. For reference, 1 cup of cooked lentils provides about 18 grams of protein compared to 14 grams in chickpeas. This is my go-to when I want a faster and protein-packed homemade falafel.

High-Protein Red Lentil Falafel

SERVES 6 • PREP TIME: 4 HOURS • COOKING TIME: 23 MINUTES

2 cups dried red lentils, rinsed well

1 cup packed fresh parsley, stems removed

¾ cup packed fresh cilantro, stems removed

1 large shallot or ¼ small red onion, roughly chopped

6 garlic cloves, minced

1 tablespoon ground cumin

2 teaspoons ground coriander

½ teaspoon ground cardamom

2 to 3 tablespoons all-purpose flour or chickpea flour, spooned and leveled

1 teaspoon baking powder

Kosher salt to taste (I use about ½ teaspoon)

Avocado oil spray or any high-heat oil

Fresh pita, hummus, and veggies, for serving

To a large mixing bowl, add the lentils and enough water to cover them by 2 inches. Cover the bowl and allow the lentils to soak for 3 hours.

Drain the lentils in a large mesh sieve and let them sit over a medium bowl for a few minutes as you prepare your remaining ingredients.

To a food processor, add the parsley, cilantro, shallot, garlic, cumin, coriander, and cardamom, then run the food processor to mince everything together. Add the lentils, 2 tablespoons of flour, the baking powder, and some salt. Run the food processor again on high in 30-second intervals, making sure to scrape down the sides as needed. Continue this process until the mixture resembles the texture of coarse sand.

Cover the mixture and place in the fridge for an hour to set.

Preheat the oven to 375°F. Line a baking sheet with parchment paper and spray with the oil.

Grab 2 to 3 tablespoons of the lentil mixture and form into a patty shape that is about ½ inch in thickness. The patties will feel soft and fragile when shaping, but this is okay. If the mixture is too wet and not holding its shape, stir another tablespoon of flour into the lentil mixture, then form again.

Place the formed patties on the prepared baking sheet. Spray the tops of the patties with more oil and then place in the oven to bake for 15 minutes. Flip and bake for an extra 5 to 8 minutes or until golden brown.

Serve with fresh pita, hummus, and fresh veggies, then enjoy!

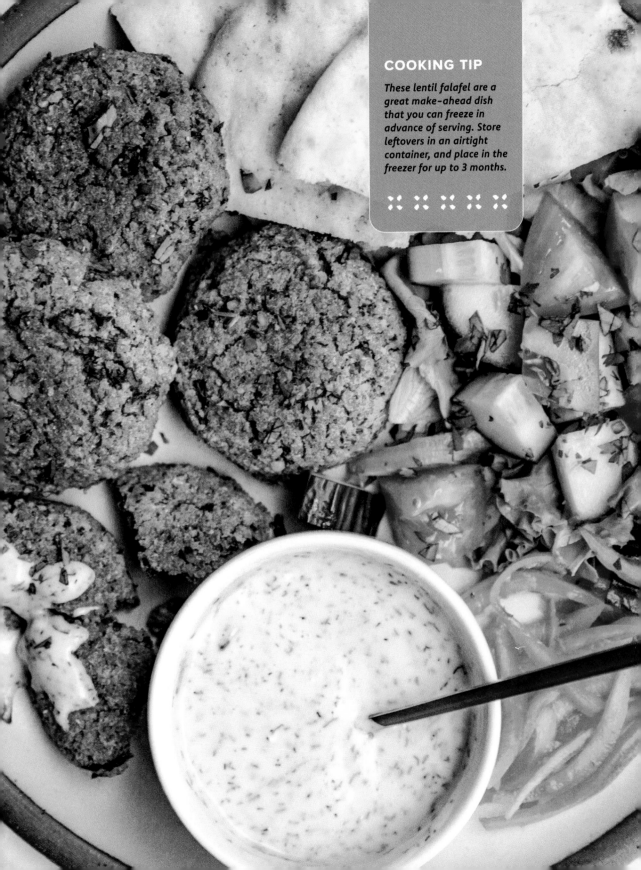

COOKING TIP

These lentil falafel are a great make-ahead dish that you can freeze in advance of serving. Store leftovers in an airtight container, and place in the freezer for up to 3 months.

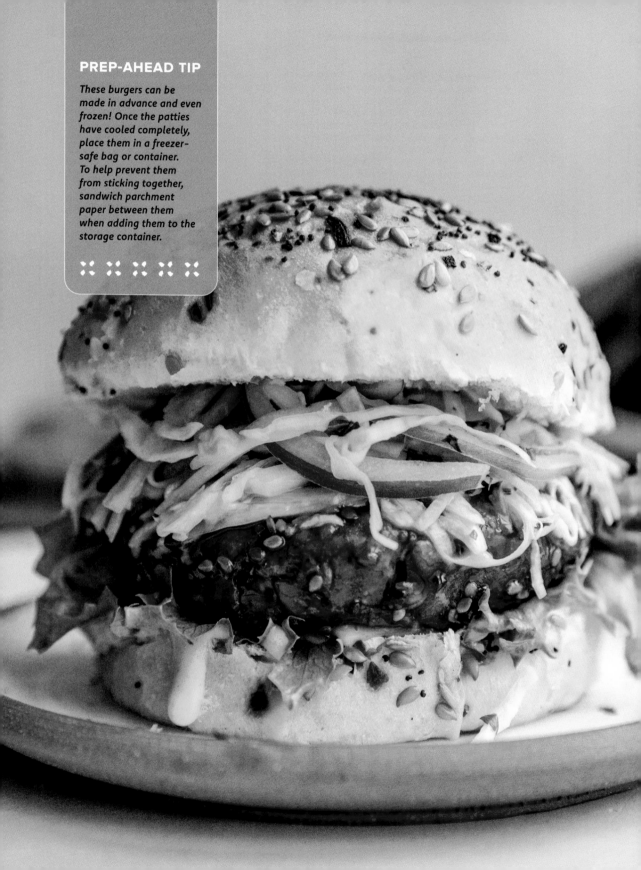

PREP-AHEAD TIP

These burgers can be made in advance and even frozen! Once the patties have cooled completely, place them in a freezer-safe bag or container. To help prevent them from sticking together, sandwich parchment paper between them when adding them to the storage container.

There is something I miss a lot from when I first went vegan, and that something is veggie burgers. It's not that they don't exist anymore, but now that a lot of great vegan meat alternatives exist, a lot of the fun and creative veggie burgers on the menu have been replaced or modified. Over the years I have figured out my own way of making these burgers better. Obviously, loading them up with flavor is essential, but also getting the right texture is key. So to help make your burgers less mushy, it's important to remove excess moisture. This is done here by patting the chickpeas dry, then giving them a quick initial roast in the oven to dry them out a little. Form your patties, and then for an extra point of flavor, baste them in a sauce you love. I did teriyaki sauce for this, but you can flex your creativity muscles and try playing around with different flavor combos you love to make the burger of your dreams, too.

Teriyaki Chickpea Burgers

SERVES 6 • PREP TIME: 15 MINUTES • COOKING TIME: 40 MINUTES

2 15-ounce cans chickpeas, drained and rinsed

2 teaspoons avocado oil, plus more as needed

1 large shallot, minced

1 Fresno chile, minced

5 garlic cloves, crushed with a garlic press

1-inch piece fresh ginger, grated

Kosher salt to taste

1/3 cup panko or fine-dried breadcrumbs

3 tablespoons all-purpose flour or chickpea flour, spooned and leveled

1/2 teaspoon five-spice powder

Pinch of white pepper

2 tablespoons natural almond butter

1 tablespoon soy sauce

1/4 cup teriyaki sauce

Burger fixings: burger buns, Easy No-Mayo Slaw (page 157), vegan mayo, and sriracha

Preheat the oven to 400°F. Line two baking sheets with parchment paper.

Place the chickpeas on a clean kitchen towel and pat dry to remove excess moisture. Transfer the chickpeas to the prepared baking sheet and spread them out into an even layer. Roast in the oven for 15 minutes.

Meanwhile, heat 2 teaspoons of oil in a medium sauté pan over medium-low heat. Once hot, add the shallot, chile, garlic, ginger, and a pinch of salt, then sauté for 2 to 3 minutes until the shallot has softened.

Allow the chickpeas and shallot mixture to cool for a few minutes before transferring them to a food processor. Add in the breadcrumbs, flour, five-spice powder, white pepper, almond butter, and soy sauce, then process until the ingredients are minced and form a dough, scraping down the sides as needed.

Scoop 1/3 cup of the chickpea mixture in your hands and shape into a 1/2-inch-thick patty. Repeat to make five more. Place the patties on a prepared baking sheet. Brush both sides of the patties with a little oil, then bake in the oven for 15 minutes.

Brush the tops of the burgers with teriyaki sauce, then flip and baste the other side. Place back in the oven for 5 to 8 minutes.

Allow the burgers to rest and cool for 8 to 10 minutes before enjoying. Serve with your favorite bun and fixings.

One of the hardest things about making more nourishing meals at home is finding the time. No one wants to be told, ""Yeah, this is good for you, but you'll need an hour to prepare it." So whenever I am asked to share an easy and quick meal, I always turn to sheet pan meals. This one is a fave because *everything* including the gnocchi cooks in a pan in the oven. Roast everything to caramelize, then toss with your pesto, and dinner is served with just a few dishes to clean.

Charred Scallion Pesto Baked Gnocchi

SERVES 4 • PREP TIME: 10 MINUTES • COOKING TIME: 30 MINUTES

1 15-ounce can chickpeas, drained and rinsed

1 teaspoon garlic powder

1 teaspoon onion powder

1 teaspoon dried oregano

1 teaspoon dried basil

3 tablespoons extra-virgin olive oil

Kosher salt and freshly ground black pepper to taste

1 head cauliflower, cut into 1-inch florets

½ medium red onion, roughly chopped

1 pound package of gnocchi

1 pint cherry tomatoes

⅓ cup Charred Scallion Pesto (page 212), plus more as needed

Preheat your oven to 425°F and line 2 large baking sheets with parchment paper.

Dry your chickpeas in a clean kitchen towel. Transfer the chickpeas to one of the prepared baking sheets and sprinkle with a ½ teaspoon each of the garlic powder, onion powder, oregano, and basil. Top with 1 tablespoon of the oil and a sprinkle of salt and pepper, then toss to evenly coat. Spread the chickpeas out into a single layer on the pan.

To a large mixing bowl, add the cauliflower, red onion, 1 tablespoon of the oil, then the remaining ½ teaspoon each garlic powder, onion powder, oregano, and basil. Season with a generous pinch of salt, toss to evenly coat, then place onto half of one of the prepared baking sheets, making sure the cauliflower pieces are placed cut side down.

To the same large bowl, add your gnocchi and tomatoes. Add the remaining 1 tablespoon of the oil along with a generous pinch of salt and pepper then toss to evenly coat. Spread the mixture out on the opposite side of the cauliflower tray, making sure everything is in an even single layer.

Roast simultaneously the tray of cauliflower and gnocchi on the bottom rack and the tray of chickpeas on the top rack, for 20 minutes. Toss the chickpeas and flip the cauliflower, then bake for an additional 10 minutes or until golden.

Add the pesto to the tray of cauliflower and gnocchi and stir well to evenly coat. Serve the cauliflower and gnocchi topped with the crispy chickpeas and extra pesto if desired.

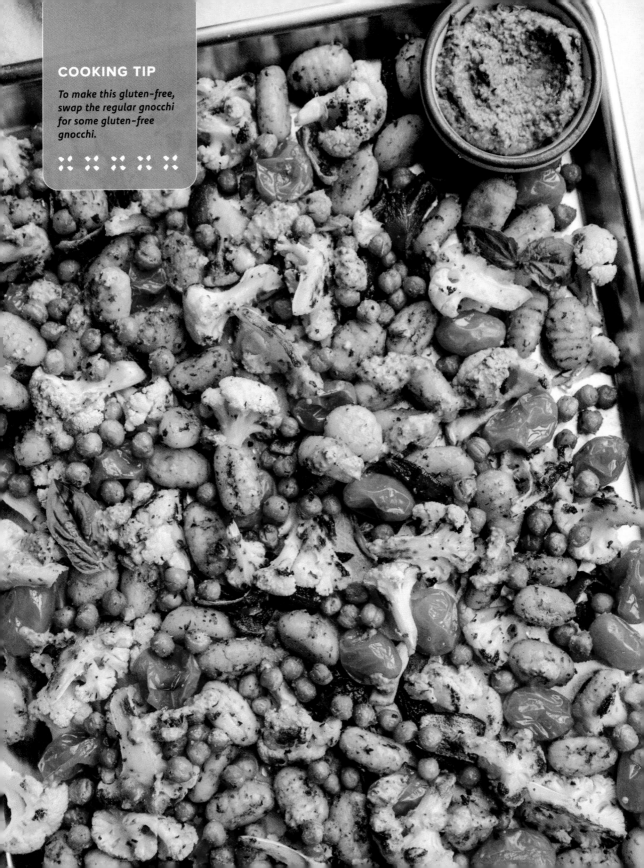

COOKING TIP

To make this gluten-free, swap the regular gnocchi for some gluten-free gnocchi.

CHAPTER 6

Let's give veggies their WELL-DESERVED flowers. These recipes put veggies as the main focus and pack them in with FLAVOR. Eating your vegetables this way will have you LOOKING FORWARD to getting in all your servings for the day.

Elevated Veggies

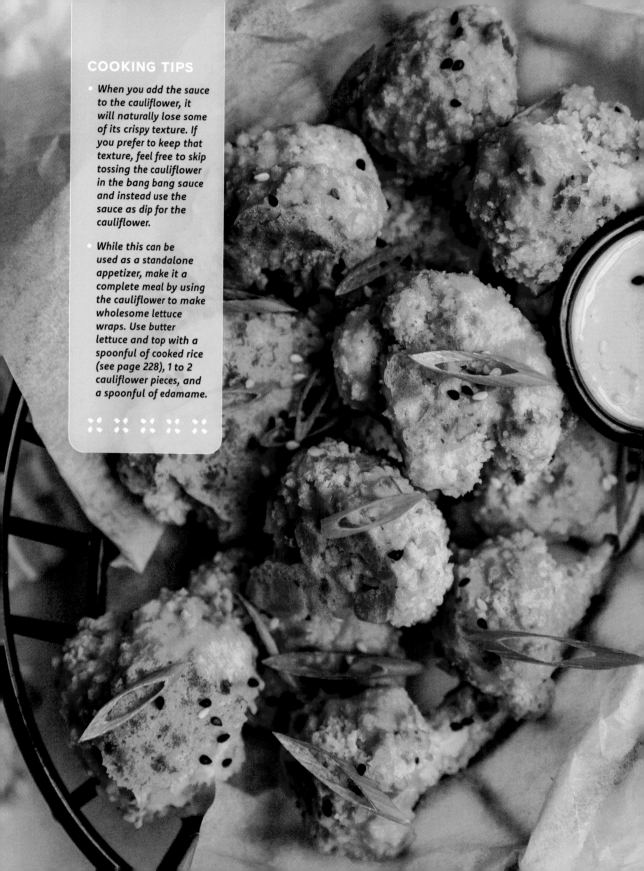

COOKING TIPS

- When you add the sauce to the cauliflower, it will naturally lose some of its crispy texture. If you prefer to keep that texture, feel free to skip tossing the cauliflower in the bang bang sauce and instead use the sauce as dip for the cauliflower.

- While this can be used as a standalone appetizer, make it a complete meal by using the cauliflower to make wholesome lettuce wraps. Use butter lettuce and top with a spoonful of cooked rice (see page 228), 1 to 2 cauliflower pieces, and a spoonful of edamame.

This is probably the cauliflower recipe I make the most. It also completely transformed my husband's opinion of cauliflower, one of his least favorite vegetables. Who would have thought just breading your cauliflower and tossing it in a delicious sauce would be enough to change that opinion quickly. But seriously, these are insanely good. They're crispy with a sweet and tangy bite. Maybe they can make you equally addicted to this humble veggie, too.

Bang Bang Cauliflower

SERVES 4 • PREP TIME: 15 MINUTES • COOKING TIME: 25 MINUTES

FOR THE CAULIFLOWER

¾ cup all-purpose flour, spooned and leveled

1 cup unsweetened almond milk

2 tablespoons nutritional yeast

1 tablespoon garlic chili sauce

½ teaspoon kosher salt

½ teaspoon freshly ground black pepper

1½ cups panko crumbs

1 teaspoon garlic powder

1 teaspoon onion powder

1 medium head cauliflower, cut into golf ball–size florets

FOR THE SAUCE

Juice of 1 lime

⅓ cup good-quality tahini (see page 59) or vegan mayonnaise

2 tablespoons garlic chili sauce

2 tablespoons maple syrup

1 teaspoon toasted sesame oil

PREPARE THE CAULIFLOWER

Preheat the oven to 425°F and line a sheet pan with parchment paper.

In a large bowl combine the flour, almond milk, nutritional yeast, chili sauce, salt, and pepper and whisk to combine.

To a separate small bowl, add the panko, garlic powder, and onion powder and whisk to combine.

Place the cauliflower florets in the batter and toss to coat evenly with a spatula. Once fully coated, take a floret and shake off any excess batter. Transfer the battered florets individually to the breadcrumb mixture and coat completely in the panko mixture.

Place the breaded cauliflower onto the prepared baking sheet, making sure that the florets have a little space between them. Once all the florets are coated, place the baking sheet in the oven for 22 minutes.

PREPARE THE SAUCE

Combine the lime juice, tahini, chili sauce, maple syrup, toasted sesame oil, and ¼ cup water in a small bowl and whisk together until smooth. If the sauce is too thick, add additional water 1 tablespoon at a time and whisk until you achieve a creamy, pourable sauce.

Add the cooked florets to a large bowl and pour over with the sauce. With a spatula, carefully toss the florets until fully coated. With tongs, place the individual florets back onto the baking sheet and return to the oven to bake for an additional 3 minutes or until the sauce has set, then enjoy.

Green beans are severely underrated! Usually the only time I ever see or hear people talk about them enthusiastically is during the holidays, but there is a world beyond green bean casserole. So, use this as your sign to be more enthusiastic about green beans all year round, especially when they can taste like this—savory, garlicky, and a little spicy. Like many vegetables, green beans provide fiber and a variety of vitamins and minerals that can help support heart health. So make that a reason to make them tasty and enjoy more of them.

Gochujang Stir-Fried Green Beans

SERVES 4 • PREP TIME: 5 MINUTES • COOKING TIME: 7 MINUTES

1 tablespoon avocado oil

12 ounces green beans, ends trimmed

1 large shallot, sliced

Kosher salt to taste

5 garlic cloves, crushed using a garlic press

1 tablespoon gochujang

1 tablespoon reduced-sodium soy sauce or coconut aminos

Sesame seeds, for serving

1 teaspoon sesame oil (optional), for serving

Heat the oil in a large heavy-bottomed skillet over medium heat. Once the oil is hot, add the green beans. Spread the green beans out in a single layer and allow to cook undisturbed for 1 to 2 minutes.

Add the shallot along with a pinch of salt, then toss together with the green beans. Continue to cook, stirring occasionally for 2 to 3 more minutes to char the green beans.

Add in the garlic, stirring constantly until fragrant, about 1 minute. Stir in the gochujang and soy sauce, then continue sautéing for 2 minutes to coat the green beans.

Serve garnished with sesame seeds and a touch of sesame oil, if desired, then enjoy.

Though it is sometimes hard to admit, I often struggle figuring out what to do with leftover veggies in the fridge. Many times in the past, I would just push these forgotten veggies farther and farther back in the fridge, only to find them weeks later, unsalvageable. This used to happen often because I just didn't have a plan for what to do with that little bit of extra something left over from a recipe. Now, I save those veggies in a bin I can see, and when I gather enough random veggies, I make veggie pancakes. They are heavily influenced by Yachaejeon (야채전), a Korean vegetable pancake that when cooked has nice crispy edges and a lovely chewy center. They are my favorite way to use up leftover veggies and prevent a lot of unnecessary food waste.

Eat the Rainbow Veggie Pancakes (Yachaejeon 야채전)

SERVES 3 • PREP TIME: 20 MINUTES • COOKING TIME: 25 MINUTES

FOR THE PANCAKE BATTER

1 cup (130g) all-purpose flour, spooned and leveled

3 tablespoons cornstarch or potato starch

2 tablespoons nutritional yeast

½ tablespoon baking powder

1 teaspoon ground ginger

2 teaspoons garlic powder

½ teaspoon kosher salt

1 cup shredded cabbage, red or green or a combination of the two

4 scallions, thinly sliced

½ red bell pepper, thinly sliced

1 small zucchini, shredded

1 small sweet potato or carrot, peeled and shredded

1 jalapeño, seeded and thinly sliced

2 tablespoons avocado oil, plus more as needed

PREPARE THE PANCAKE BATTER

To a large mixing bowl add the flour, cornstarch, nutritional yeast, baking powder, ground ginger, garlic powder, and salt and whisk together to combine.

Pour in 1 cup water and whisk together to form a thick batter.

Add in the cabbage, scallions, bell pepper, zucchini, sweet potato, and jalapeño (this is about four cups of shredded vegetables) and fold them into the batter until completely coated.

Heat a medium nonstick pan over medium heat with 1 tablespoon of the oil. Once the oil is hot, swirl it around in the pan, then add a generous scoop of the vegetable batter in the center and spread it out as thinly and evenly as possible over the surface of the pan. Fill in any holes that appear with a little more of the vegetable batter as needed.

Cook the pancake undisturbed for about 4 minutes or until the batter starts to dry up on top and looks golden brown around the edges. Carefully flip the pancake and cook on the other side for about 4 minutes. Lower the heat, flip your pancake again, and cook for 2 to 3 minutes more. Transfer the pancake to a wire rack, heat more oil in the pan, and repeat this process with the remaining batter.

Recipe continues

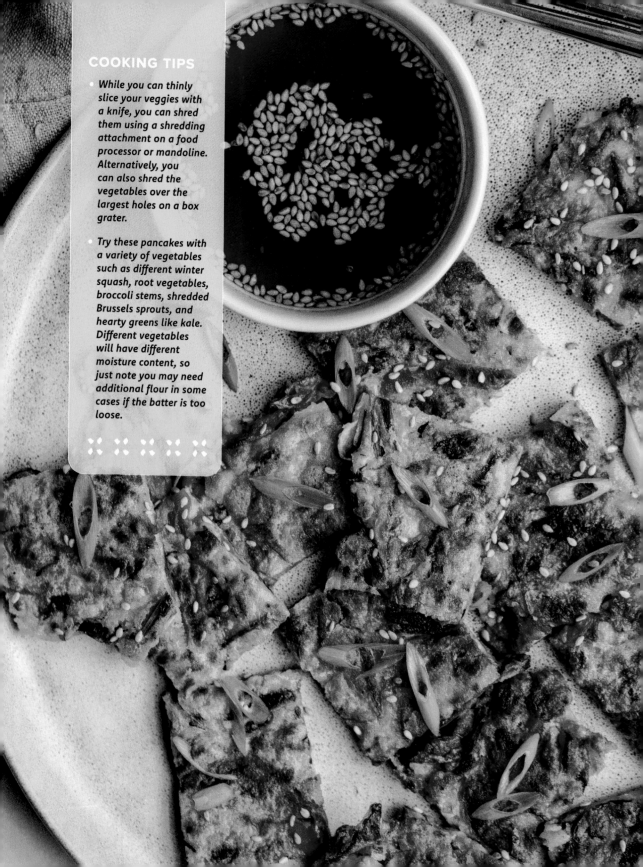

COOKING TIPS

- While you can thinly slice your veggies with a knife, you can shred them using a shredding attachment on a food processor or mandoline. Alternatively, you can also shred the vegetables over the largest holes on a box grater.

- Try these pancakes with a variety of vegetables such as different winter squash, root vegetables, broccoli stems, shredded Brussels sprouts, and hearty greens like kale. Different vegetables will have different moisture content, so just note you may need additional flour in some cases if the batter is too loose.

2 teaspoons tamari

2 teaspoons rice vinegar

2 teaspoons maple syrup

1 teaspoon sriracha

1 teaspoon toasted sesame seeds

PREPARE THE DIPPING SAUCE

To a small bowl, add the tamari, vinegar, maple syrup, sriracha, and sesame seeds and mix together, then set aside.

TO SERVE AND STORE

Slice your pancake into 2-inch pieces using a sharp knife and serve with the dipping sauce.

If you have extra pancakes you don't plan on eating right away, store them in an airtight resealable bag in the fridge for 5 days. To reheat, place the pancake back in the pan with a little oil and warm through for a few minutes on each side until they are crisp around the edges again. You can also freeze them and reheat them in the air fryer for 5 minutes at 375°F until nice and crisp, too.

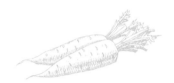

Brussels sprouts used to be one of the vegetables I heard the most complaints about from friends, family, and clients. Luckily, they are starting to gain more appreciation and love. And perhaps a lot of that is thanks to preparations that go beyond just boiling them. Searing them and experimenting with flavors that better complement this cruciferous vegetable has all made a big difference. And with my own experimenting, I find that I really love pairing them with salty sweet flavors to balance some of their natural bitterness and bring out more of their umami flavors. This citrusy, sticky sauce is a must try with them. As the sauce reduces, you get this lovely sticky glaze over them that will make you want to eat the whole batch in one go.

Braised Orange Ginger Brussels Sprouts

SERVES 4 • PREP TIME: 10 MINUTES • COOKING TIME: 15 MINUTES

2 teaspoons yellow or white miso paste

1 tablespoon tamari (see page xli)

1 tablespoon maple syrup

½ tablespoon rice vinegar

½-inch piece fresh ginger, grated

3 garlic cloves, minced

3 tablespoons orange juice

1 tablespoon avocado oil

12 ounces Brussels sprouts, trimmed and halved

In a small bowl, combine the miso paste, tamari, maple syrup, vinegar, ginger, garlic, and orange juice, as well as ⅓ cup water, then whisk together, making sure the miso paste is fully dissolved.

Heat a large skillet with the oil over medium-low heat. Once the oil is hot, add the Brussels sprouts to the pan cut side down. Allow the Brussels sprouts to cook undisturbed for 3 to 4 minutes or until golden brown in color.

Flip the Brussels sprouts on their back and cook for an additional 3 minutes to sear.

Lower the heat on the stovetop, then pour in the sauce. Allow it to come to a simmer while tossing the Brussels sprouts cut side down again. As the sauce reduces and thickens, start tossing the Brussels sprouts to fully coat them in the sauce. Once the Brussels sprouts are nice and sticky, remove from the heat and serve.

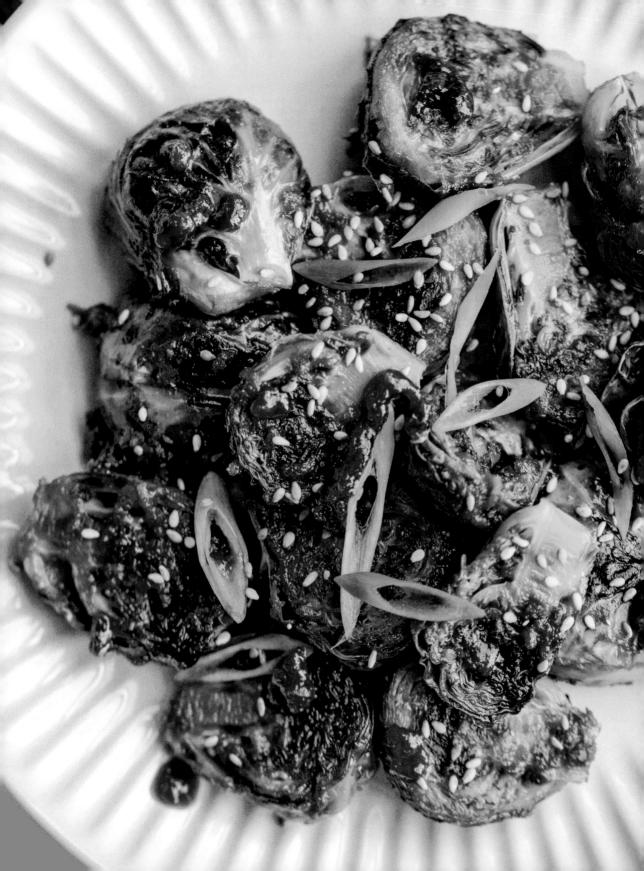

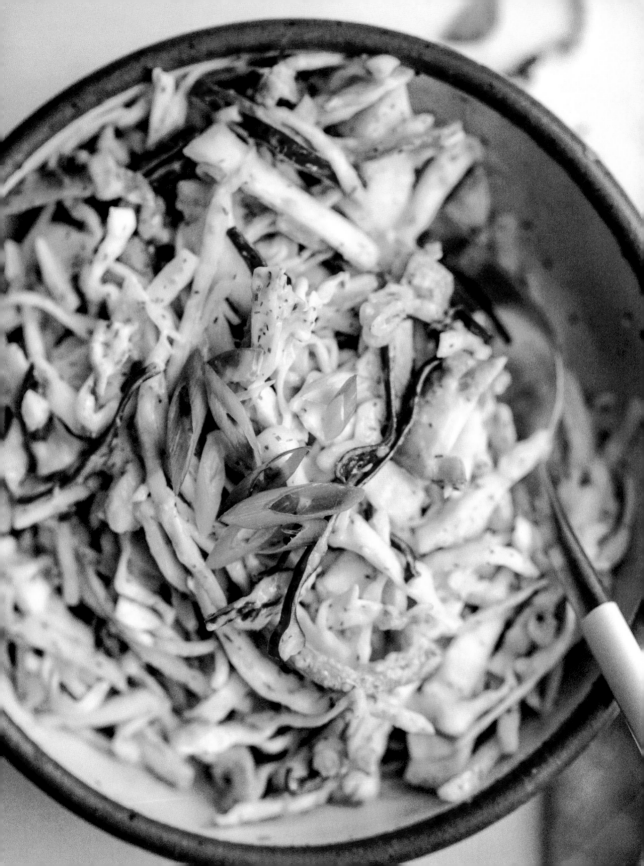

If cabbage is prepared this exact way for me, I could very happily and easily eat a whole head of cabbage. Okay, a small head of cabbage, but nonetheless, I stand by how good this is. And while there is no mayo involved in this dreamy slaw, we are still able to make a creamy and delicious dressing using plant-based ingredients. You get the perfect amount of tang from the yogurt, richness from the avocado, and a lot of freshness from the dill. And it's super easy to put together, which is probably why you'll find me at most times of the year with a big tub of this somewhere in my fridge.

Easy No-Mayo Slaw

SERVES 4 • PREP TIME: 15 MINUTES

FOR THE SLAW

4 cups green cabbage, shredded

½ cup red cabbage, shredded

1 jalapeño, seeded and thinly sliced

3 scallions, thinly sliced

Kosher salt to taste

FOR THE LEMON-DILL DRESSING

½ ripe avocado

½ cup plain unsweetened plant-based yogurt

¼ cup fresh dill, stems removed

1 tablespoon capers

1 garlic clove, grated

Juice of 1 lemon

1 tablespoon apple cider vinegar

1 teaspoon Dijon mustard

PREPARE THE SLAW

To a large mixing bowl, add the green and red cabbage, jalapeño, scallions, and a pinch of salt. Give the slaw a mix then set aside to make the dressing.

PREPARE THE LEMON-DILL DRESSING

To a mini food processor, add the avocado, yogurt, dill, capers, garlic, lemon juice, vinegar, mustard, and ¼ teaspoon salt and blend on high until the dressing is mostly smooth and the dill is finely minced.

Pour the dressing over the slaw and toss together to evenly coat the vegetables. Taste and adjust with more salt as needed. Store leftover slaw in an airtight container in the fridge for up to 3 days.

Eggplant is a very underappreciated vegetable. So let's work on making it crave-worthy in the best possible way. This eggplant gets perfectly tender in the oven, then is roasted with a peanut-miso glaze. The preparation is based on a classic Japanese recipe, Nasu no Miso Dengaku (茄子の味噌田楽) or miso-glazed eggplant. Typically, the eggplant is grilled, then brushed with a sweet miso glaze. However, with this preparation we are using the oven and broiler to achieve a fantastic tender melt-in-your-mouth texture. Less mess and you can cook all the eggplant at the same time in one batch.

Roasted Peanut Miso Eggplant

SERVES 3 • PREP TIME: 15 MINUTES • COOKING TIME: 20 MINUTES

2 tablespoons natural peanut butter

1 tablespoon yellow or white miso paste

2 garlic cloves, crushed with a garlic press

1 tablespoon maple syrup

1 tablespoon mirin

3 small eggplant (you can use purple, graffiti, or Chinese eggplant)

Kosher salt to taste

1 tablespoon avocado oil

1 tablespoon tamari

FOR SERVING

Toasted sesame oil

Toasted sesame seeds

Sliced scallions

Preheat the oven to 425°F. Line a baking sheet with parchment paper.

To a small bowl add the peanut butter, miso paste, garlic, maple syrup, mirin, and 1 tablespoon water, then whisk together until smooth.

Cut off the top of each eggplant and then cut the eggplant in half lengthwise. With a sharp knife, score the flesh of the eggplant diagonally across the length of the eggplant. Then score the eggplant in the opposite direction to create a tight crisscross pattern. When scoring the eggplant, make sure you are cutting about 2/3 of the way into the flesh.

Fill a large bowl with water and a generous pinch of salt. Soak the eggplant in the water for 10 minutes to help remove any astringency from the eggplant. Remove the eggplant from the bowl and rinse well under running water. Blot the eggplant dry using a kitchen towel, then place on the prepared baking sheet cut side up.

In a small bowl, mix the avocado oil and tamari together, then brush it over the flesh of the eggplant halves and place the eggplant cut side down on the baking sheet. Bake the eggplant in the oven for 20 minutes or until the eggplant is tender.

Remove the eggplant from the oven and turn them over so the eggplant is facing cut side up. Brush the peanut sauce generously to coat the surface of the eggplant completely.

Place the eggplant back in the oven and set to broil. Broil the eggplant for 4 to 5 minutes or until the sauce begins to bubble on top. Remove from the oven.

TO SERVE

Serve topped with a drizzle of sesame oil, toasted sesame seeds, and fresh sliced scallions.

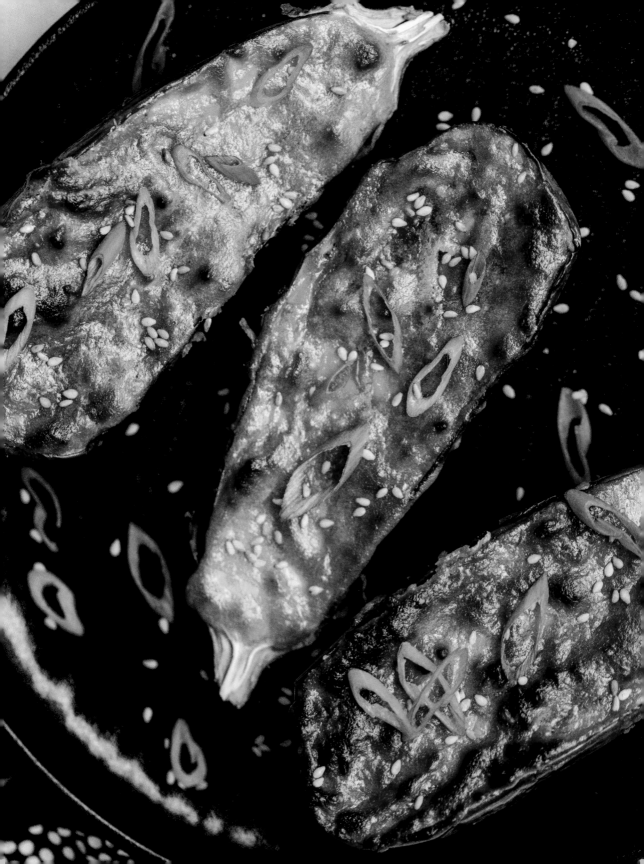

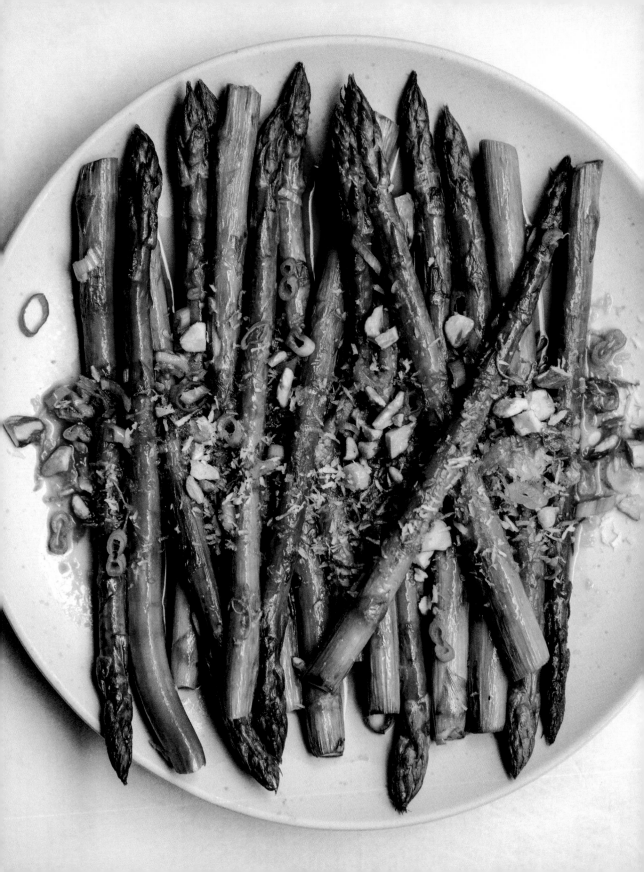

Asparagus is one of my favorite vegetables because it typically involves the least amount of chopping when you're feeling lazy. It's also really good when cooked right. Honestly, just searing or roasting it in some oil and finishing it with a pinch of salt is enough for me to enjoy it. However, you can truly elevate asparagus and make it something special with an additional savory sauce and some fun toppings. Both take no more than 5 minutes to make. So once your asparagus is nice and blistered, drizzle the sauce on top and sprinkle on the pistachio-and-coconut mix to create the ultimate side.

Seared Asparagus with Pistachio Coconut Relish

SERVES 4 • PREP TIME: 5 MINUTES • COOKING TIME: 5 MINUTES

2 tablespoons pistachios, roughly chopped

1 tablespoon unsweetened shredded coconut flakes

Zest and juice of ½ lime

Kosher salt to taste

1 tablespoon tamari

1 tablespoon sweet chili sauce

2 teaspoons maple syrup

1 teaspoon sesame oil

1 tablespoon extra-virgin olive oil

12 ounces asparagus, woody stems cut and discarded

1 scallion, thinly sliced

To a small bowl, add the pistachios, coconut flakes, lime zest, and a pinch of salt. Mix together until well combined.

In a separate small bowl, combine the tamari, chili sauce, maple syrup, lime juice, and sesame oil, then whisk together.

Heat a large skillet with the olive oil over medium heat. Add the asparagus spears to the pan and spread them out in a single layer so most of the asparagus is touching the bottom of the pan. Cook undisturbed for 2 minutes, then give them a toss, spread them out again, and cook undisturbed for another 2 minutes. Add the scallion and sauté with the asparagus for an additional minute until the asparagus is bright green. Sprinkle the asparagus with a pinch of salt, then transfer to a serving dish.

Drizzle the sauce over top of the asparagus, then sprinkle the pistachio-and-coconut mix on top and serve.

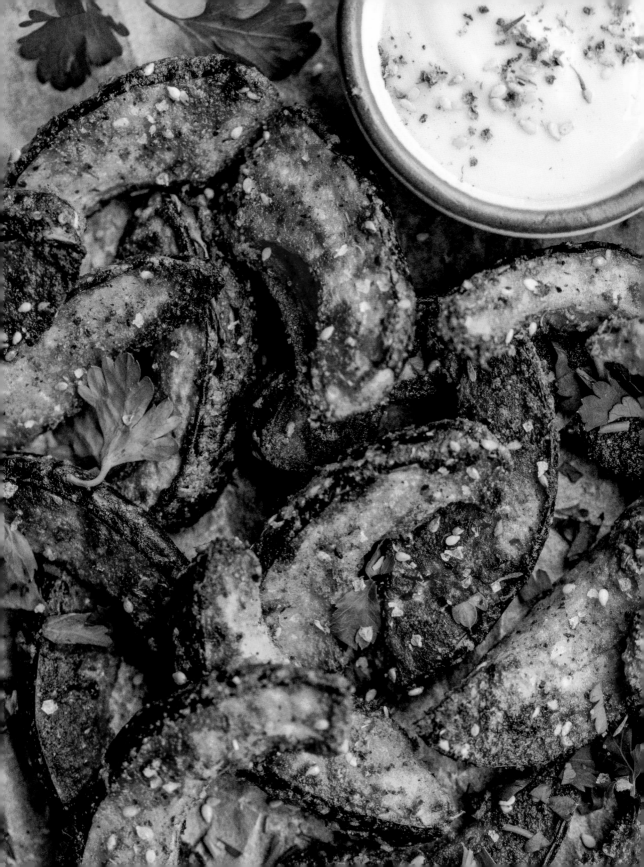

I always want to celebrate how amazing vegetables and fruits can be. You just have to keep an open mind and maintain a well-stocked spice cabinet. Spices and herbs can truly transform the least exciting vegetables into something special. One spice I have grown to love over the years is za'atar. It's a Middle Eastern spice blend used in Levantine cuisine, and while the preparation of this spice can vary from one country to another, most blends contain a combination of dried sumac, toasted sesame seeds, and other dry herbs. Za'atar adds a citrusy, savory, and earthy flavor that goes especially well with vegetables. So using it to coat some acorn squash came to me as a no-brainer. You get a flavorful crusty exterior and a tender soft inside that will make you want to happily eat a whole acorn squash by yourself.

Za'atar Roasted Acorn Squash Wedges

SERVES 2 TO 3 • PREP TIME: 5 MINUTES • COOKING TIME: 35 MINUTES

1 small acorn squash (1 pound)

1½ tablespoons avocado oil

1 tablespoon cornstarch

1 tablespoon nutritional yeast

2 teaspoons za'atar

1 teaspoon garlic powder

Kosher salt to taste

Maple Dijon Dressing (page 205), for serving

Preheat the oven to 425°F. Line a baking sheet with parchment paper.

With a sharp knife, carefully cut the ends of the acorn squash off, then cut it in half lengthwise to expose the seeds. With a spoon, scoop out the seeds, then cut the squash into 1-inch-thick wedges.

To a large bowl, add the squash wedges and top with the oil, cornstarch, nutritional yeast, za'atar, garlic powder, and a generous pinch of salt. Toss the wedges in the mixture until evenly coated. If using a larger squash, feel free to use a little more oil to coat as needed.

Transfer the wedges to the prepared baking sheet and spread them out in a single layer with space between the wedges. Place the tray in the oven on the bottom rack and bake for 25 minutes.

Salt the wedges and flip, then bake for another 10 minutes or until brown on both sides.

Sprinkle with extra salt if desired, then serve immediately with your favorite dip like some Maple Dijon Dressing and enjoy!

This might sound weird, but have you ever grilled your lettuce? I promise, it tastes much better than you think, and it's a really great way to get in more veggies. So what does grilling your greens actually do? For the short time the lettuce cooks, it helps to caramelize and char the greens to give them more umami flavor in every crispy bite. Try it once, and you'll be hooked.

Grilled Maple Dijon Lettuce

SERVES 2 TO 3 • PREP TIME: 5 MINUTES • COOKING TIME: 8 MINUTES

¼ cup sliced almonds

1 tablespoon avocado oil

¼ teaspoon lemon pepper

½ teaspoon ground coriander

¼ teaspoon red pepper flakes

Zest of 1 small lemon

Kosher salt to taste

Freshly ground black pepper to taste

2 small heads romaine hearts, cut in half lengthwise

½ cup cherry tomatoes, halved

Maple Dijon Dressing (page 205), for serving

Place a small sauté pan over medium-low heat. Once hot, add the almond slices and stir occasionally for 3 to 5 minutes until golden in color. Remove from the heat, then transfer the almonds to a small bowl and set aside.

In a separate small bowl combine the oil, lemon pepper, coriander, red pepper flakes, lemon zest, and a pinch of salt and pepper. Whisk to combine, then brush onto the cut side of each romaine heart.

Heat a grill pan over medium-high heat, then place the romaine hearts in the pan cut side down. Allow the lettuce to cook for 1 to 2 minutes until grill marks appear, then remove from the pan and place on a serving platter.

Top the platter with cherry tomatoes and toasted almonds, then drizzle a few spoons of the Maple Dijon Dressing over top and serve.

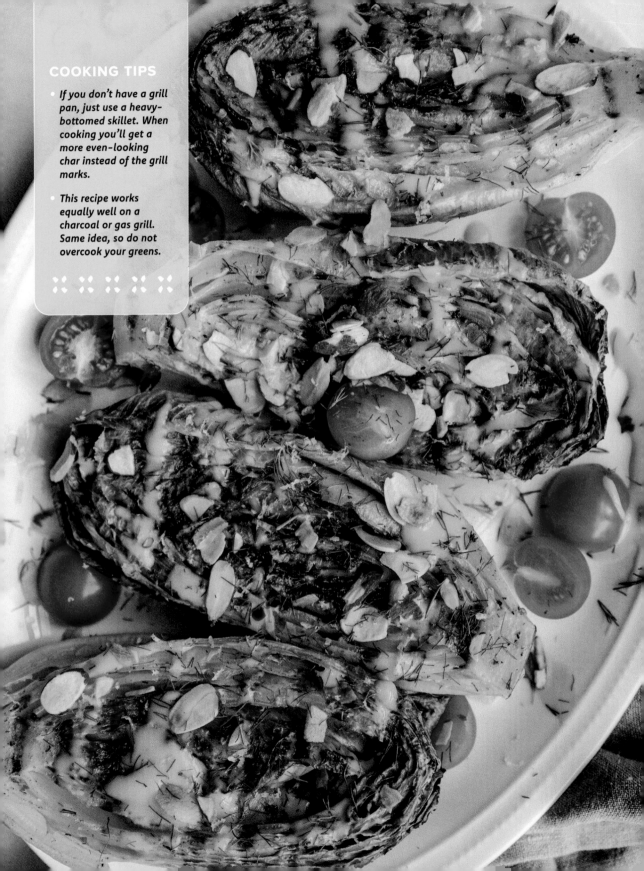

COOKING TIPS

- *If you don't have a grill pan, just use a heavy-bottomed skillet. When cooking you'll get a more even-looking char instead of the grill marks.*

- *This recipe works equally well on a charcoal or gas grill. Same idea, so do not overcook your greens.*

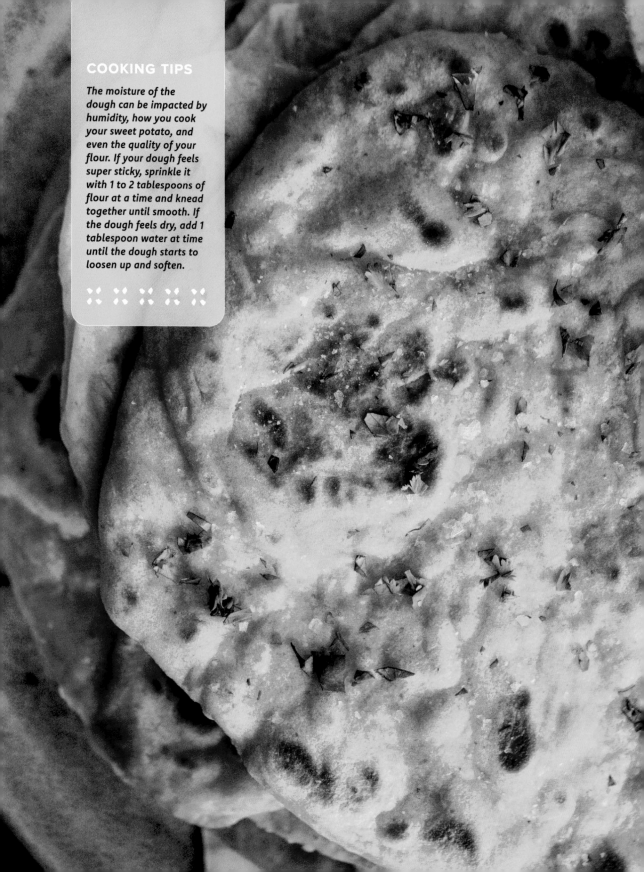

COOKING TIPS

The moisture of the dough can be impacted by humidity, how you cook your sweet potato, and even the quality of your flour. If your dough feels super sticky, sprinkle it with 1 to 2 tablespoons of flour at a time and knead together until smooth. If the dough feels dry, add 1 tablespoon water at time until the dough starts to loosen up and soften.

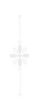

What if I told you that you can have superfluffy and tasty flatbread that is not only faster than the average yeasted flatbread but also more nourishing? Excited, right? Honestly, I was and it's not that difficult to make. No yeast needed, and we get the fluffiness from both the yogurt and sweet potato. The yogurt has active cultures that help give some yeastlike activity to our bread while the sweet potato gives us a softer dough that is loaded with beta-carotene, vitamin C, and potassium. Truly, I am always amazed when you can create food that you love that also loves you back.

Sweet Potato Flatbread

SERVES 8 • PREP TIME: 80 MINUTES • COOKING TIME: 30 MINUTES

1 sweet potato or
½ cup pumpkin puree

2 cups (270 g) all-purpose flour, spooned and leveled, plus more as needed

2 teaspoons baking powder

½ teaspoon kosher salt, plus more to taste

½ cup plain unsweetened plant-based yogurt

3 tablespoons avocado oil, plus more as needed

Preheat the oven to 400°F. Choose a large sweet potato, rinse it well, and poke the surface a few times with a fork. Roast your sweet potato on a baking sheet for 1 hour, or until softened and easy to mash. Allow to cool, cut in half, and scoop out the flesh and mash really well. You can also microwave the potato on a microwave-safe plate for 4 minutes per side or until fork-tender to make this faster.

To a medium mixing bowl, add the flour, baking powder, and salt, then whisk to combine.

Add ½ cup (140 g) mashed sweet potato and yogurt, then fold them into the dry ingredients to form a dough ball. Knead the dough a few times with your hands until the dough is nice and smooth.

If the dough is too wet, add a tablespoon of flour at a time until the dough is smooth. Place the dough back in the bowl and cover and allow to rest for 20 minutes.

Divide the dough into 8 equal pieces. Round the dough balls and place 1 dough ball on a clean, flat, well-floured surface and keep the remaining dough balls covered. Roll out each dough ball into a thin circle.

Heat a large non-stick skillet over medium heat and brush with 2 teaspoons of oil to lightly coat the pan. Add the rolled out dough and allow to cook undisturbed for 2 minutes or until you notice some bubbles forming in the dough. Flip and repeat the process, cooking on the other side for 2 to 3 minutes until evenly cooked. Optional, but you can brush both sides of the cooked flatbread with a little more oil, then transfer to a plate and sprinkle with a pinch of salt while it is still warm. Repeat this process with the remaining dough balls.

Did you know that frozen veggies can be more nutritious than the fresh veggies at your supermarket? Frozen produce is harvested at the peak of ripeness before being frozen, which helps preserve nutrients. Beyond being a great source of nutrition, they are also incredibly convenient. You can use them straight from their package with no cleaning or chopping required, and you don't have to worry about them spoiling in the freezer.

Now, if you are looking to utilize these frozen gems, it's important to note that frozen vegetables can lead to mushy results if not cooked properly. Cooking frozen vegetables is a big thing I taught during my community cooking classes. The secret is searing them in a dry pan first before sautéing with your oil and seasonings.

How to Make Frozen Veggies Taste Amazing

SERVES 3 TO 4 • PREP TIME: 5 MINUTES • COOKING TIME: 15 MINUTES

1 pound frozen vegetables of choice (I like using a mix of broccoli florets and cauliflower, but any vegetable or medley will do)

1 tablespoon extra-virgin olive oil

2 garlic cloves, minced

Kosher salt to taste

Freshly ground black pepper to taste

Fresh cilantro leaves or parsley, minced, for serving

Heat a large heavy-bottomed skillet over medium heat. Once the pan is hot, add the frozen vegetables and spread them out in a single layer in the pan. If there are pieces that have a flat edge, place them flat side down in the pan.

Allow the vegetables to cook undisturbed for 3 to 5 minutes to sear. Give the vegetables a flip when you start to see the vegetables browning, then cook again undisturbed for 3 to 5 minutes. Continue to sauté them in the pan until the vegetables have released most of their water.

Lower the heat to medium-low, then add in the oil and toss to coat. Add the minced garlic along and a generous pinch of salt and pepper, then sauté together until fragrant, about 2 minutes.

Remove from the heat and garnish with cilantro or parsley as desired before serving.

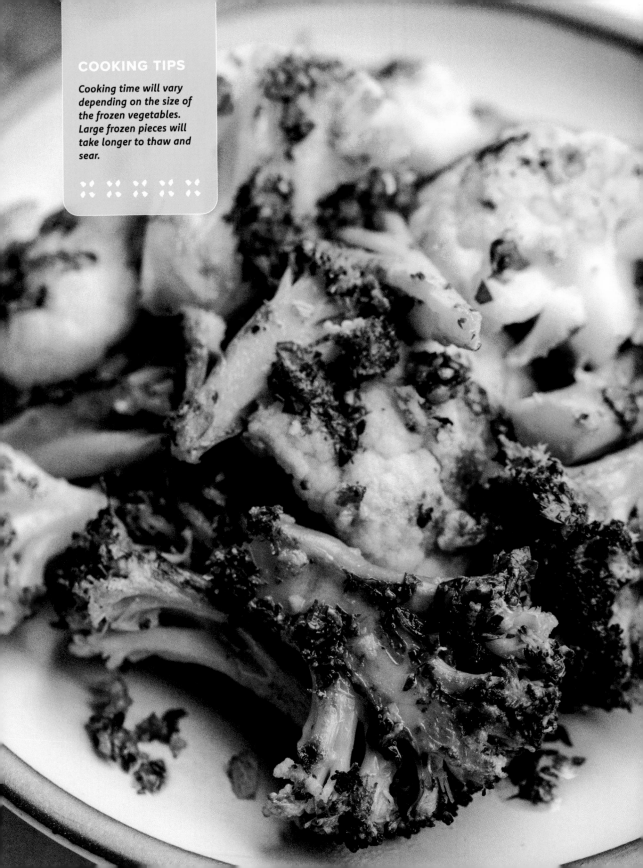

COOKING TIPS

Cooking time will vary depending on the size of the frozen vegetables. Large frozen pieces will take longer to thaw and sear.

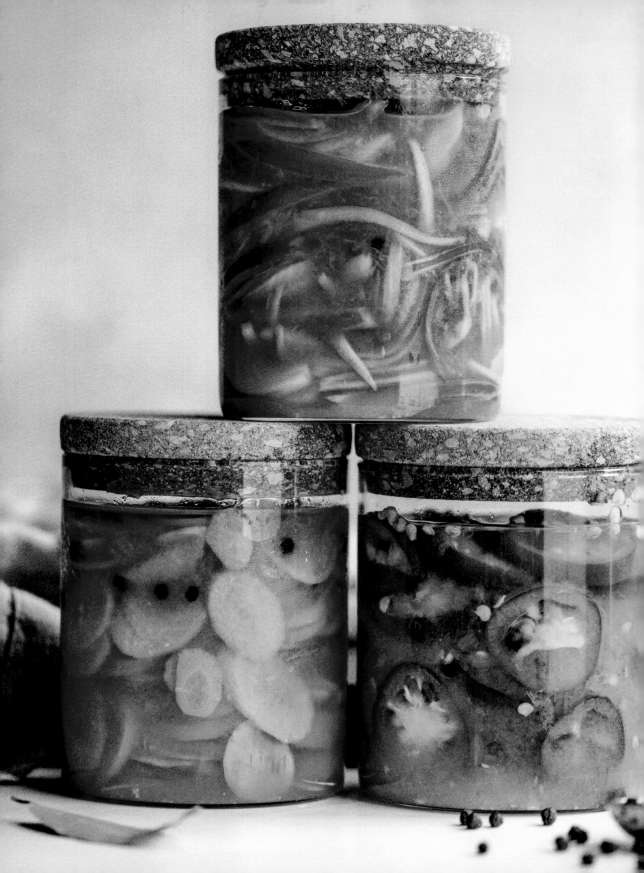

Here's a fantastic way to get the most use out of your veggies, especially the extra veggies that you don't know what to do with and don't want to have spoil. Pickling, even quick-pickling, can help extend the life of certain vegetables. Here are a few quick-pickling recipes I use frequently. Once made, you can use them as a way to add some crunch and zing to any bowl.

Pickled Vegetables

Easy Pickled Jalapeños

PREP TIME: 10 MINUTES • COOKING TIME: 8 MINUTES

I love jalapeños, but pickled jalapeños have an extra-special place in my heart. They give you a little crunch and heat that pairs perfectly with any bowl to liven it up. Surprisingly, they are cheap and super easy to make yourself. This batch in particular uses more citrus than vinegar to cure them. Using this method makes them taste delicious and maintain crunch.

3 to 4 jalapeños, sliced

Juice of 1 lime, about 3 tablespoons

Juice of 1 lemon, about 4 tablespoons

Juice of ½ orange, about 4 tablespoons

1 tablespoon vinegar

½ teaspoon kosher salt

½ teaspoon black peppercorns

1 bay leaf

Heat a medium, dry skillet over medium heat. When hot, add the jalapeños and spread them out in an even layer and cook for 1 to 2 minutes undisturbed.

Give the slices a toss and continue to cook for 3 to 4 minutes, stirring occasionally until slightly softened.

Transfer the jalapeños to a sterile 16-ounce glass jar, then cover with the lime, lemon, and orange juices. Add the vinegar, salt, and peppercorns. Stir well and press the jalapeños down into the juice, wedge in the bay leaf, and seal the jar. If the jalapeños are not completely covered in the juice, add additional boiling water as needed.

Allow the jar to cool completely then place in the fridge overnight or for at least 8 hours before enjoying. Store in the fridge for up to 2 weeks, just make sure to always use clean utensils when removing jalapeños from the jar.

Pickled Red Onions

PREP TIME: 5 MINUTES

This is by far the pickle recipe I make most. Pickled onions can literally go on everything and make everything infinitely better. Now, this preparation is a little different than most. The solution that the onions sit in is made primarily of citrus juice, which mimics the way my mom would normally make quick pickled onions growing up. The citrus juice "cooks" the onion similarly to normal vinegar solutions and tastes so much better in my humble opinion.

1 medium red onion, thinly sliced

3/4 teaspoon kosher salt

1/2 teaspoon black peppercorns

1 bay leaf

Juice of 1 lemon, about 4 tablespoons

Juice of 1 lime, about 3 tablespoons

Juice of 1/2 orange, about 4 tablespoons

1 tablespoon apple cider vinegar

To a sterile 16-ounce jar, add the onion slices. Sprinkle with the salt and add the peppercorns and bay leaf.

Pour over the lemon, lime, and orange juices and the vinegar. Do note, the onions do not need to be fully submerged in the solution. They will shrink down in size as they soften.

Seal the jar, give it a good shake to coat, then place in the fridge for 30 minutes. Give the jar another shake, then allow to continue softening for 1 to 2 hours before using. Store in the fridge for up to 2 weeks, just make sure to always use clean utensils when removing onions from the jar.

COOKING TIPS

If you are uncomfortable using a knife, use a mandoline slicer. Make sure to always use a protective glove or guard when operating a mandoline to protect your precious fingers.

Pickled Carrots and Radishes

PREP TIME: **15 MINUTES**

Sometimes a bowl or sandwich needs a little tang and crunch. These pickled carrots and radishes do both! Easy to make in advance for the week and a great way to get some extra vegetables into your meals without having to do extra cooking.

2 medium carrots, thinly sliced into coins

4 radishes, thinly sliced into coins

¾ teaspoon kosher salt

½ teaspoon black peppercorns

1 bay leaf

¼ teaspoon red pepper flakes

Juice of 1 lime, about 3 tablespoons

Juice of 1 lemon, about 4 tablespoons

Juice of 1 orange, about ¼ cup juice

3 tablespoons rice vinegar

In a 16-ounce sterile jar, layer the sliced carrots and radishes and sprinkle salt between the layers. Allow the salted carrots and radishes to sit for 30 minutes.

Add the peppercorns, bay leaf, and red pepper flakes, then pour in the lime, lemon, and orange juices and the vinegar. Seal the jar and give it a gentle shake to combine.

Place in the fridge for 12 to 24 hours before enjoying. Store in the fridge for up to 2 weeks, just make sure to always use clean utensils when removing veggies from the jar.

COOKING TIP

If the liquid doesn't fill all the way to the top, just add some boiling water from a tea kettle to cover. Allow to fully cool before sealing and placing in the fridge.

CHAPTER 7

Snacks and sweets absolutely HAVE A PLACE at the table. These are for the times you feel you need SOMETHING EXTRA to satisfy you after or between meals. Even TREATS CAN DELIVER on your nutrition goals.

Snacks & Sweets

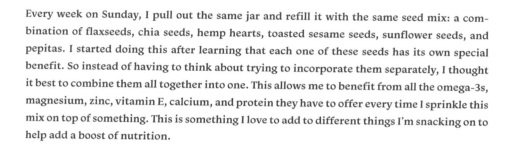

Every week on Sunday, I pull out the same jar and refill it with the same seed mix: a combination of flaxseeds, chia seeds, hemp hearts, toasted sesame seeds, sunflower seeds, and pepitas. I started doing this after learning that each one of these seeds has its own special benefit. So instead of having to think about trying to incorporate them separately, I thought it best to combine them all together into one. This allows me to benefit from all the omega-3s, magnesium, zinc, vitamin E, calcium, and protein they have to offer every time I sprinkle this mix on top of something. This is something I love to add to different things I'm snacking on to help add a boost of nutrition.

Super Seed Mix

MAKES 32 1-OUNCE SERVINGS • PREP TIME: 5 MINUTES

½ cup pepitas

½ cup sunflower seeds

¼ cup flaxseeds, ground

¼ cup chia seeds, ground

¼ cup hemp hearts

2 tablespoons toasted sesame seeds

Add the pepitas, sunflower seeds, flaxseeds, chia seeds, hemp hearts, and sesame seeds to an airtight jar and shake or stir well to evenly combine.

Place in the fridge where it can be stored for up 6 months. Shake or stir well each time before use.

Feel free to make additions to this seed-mix base to change it up. Mix in some toasted coconut flakes and cacao nibs to stir into your oats, or go the savory route and add fortified nutritional yeast for a boost in B12 and some umami flavor that goes great sprinkled over your favorite salad.

HOW TO USE

For some snack ideas using this mix: try sprinkling overtop a bowl of your favorite yogurt and fruit, mixing in with your favorite nut or seed butter to spread on top of toast or stuffed into dates, topping chia pudding for some texture, or adding into trail mix or granola.

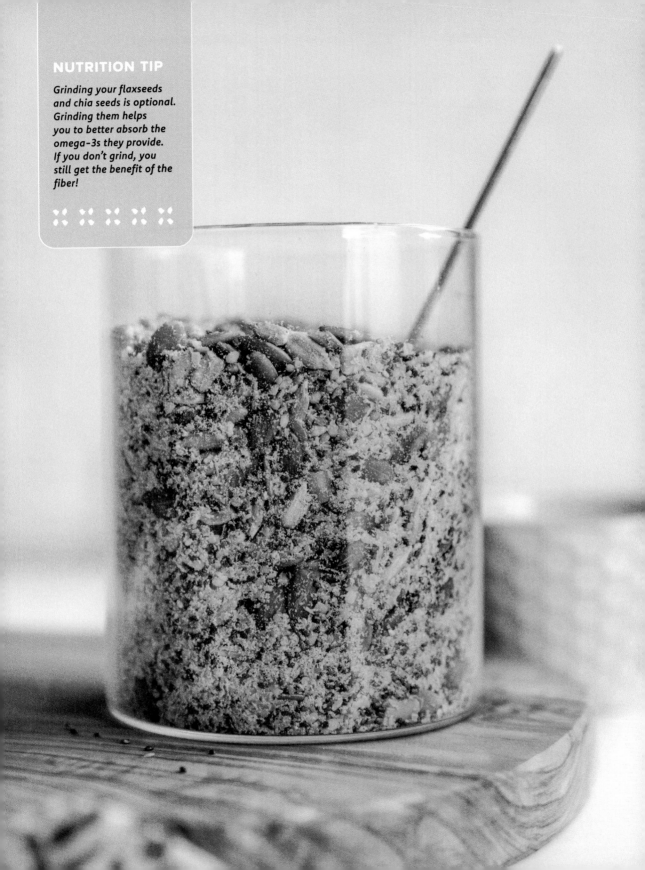

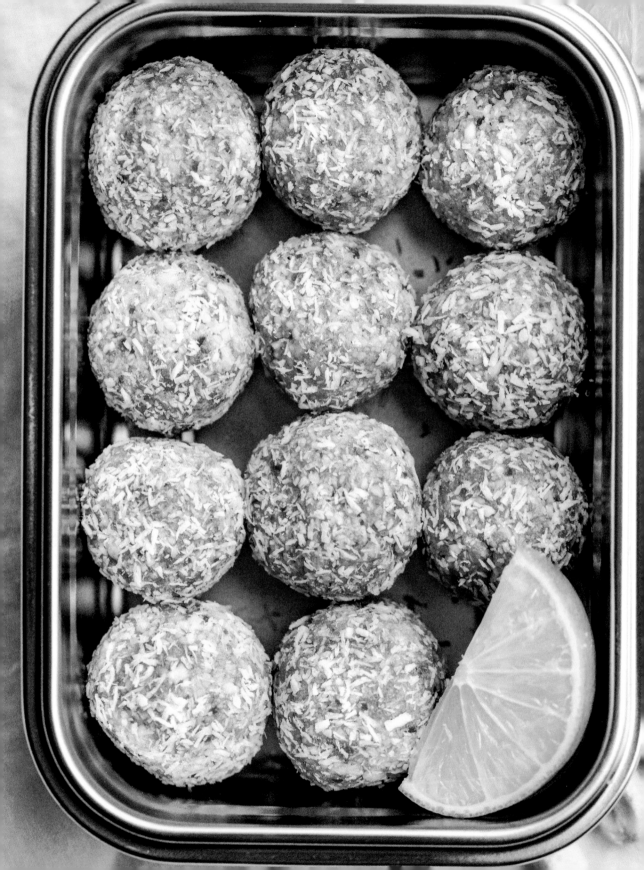

I'm a big—scratch that—HUGE fan of energy bites. I have been making a version of them ever since my intern days, and they never get old. They always hit the spot for me, and I find that amazing considering how wholesome the ingredients are. These ones in particular are a favorite thanks to the combination of lime and cardamom that adds a layer of brightness and warmth to every bite. And if you can manage not to eat the whole batch in one go, these make for a perfect prep-ahead snack for when the munchies hit.

Coconut Lime Energy Bites

MAKES 12 ENERGY BITES • PREP TIME: 20 MINUTES

¾ cup unsweetened shredded coconut flakes

1 cup raw cashews

½ cup Medjool dates, pits removed

2 tablespoons canned coconut milk or maple syrup

Zest of 1 lime

1 teaspoon ground cinnamon

½ teaspoon ground cardamom

¼ teaspoon kosher salt

To a food processor, add ½ cup shredded coconut, then the cashews, dates, coconut milk, lime zest, cinnamon, cardamom, and salt. Start by pulsing the ingredients to combine, then process on high for 1 to 2 minutes until the ingredients hold their shape when molded together with your hands.

Place the remaining ¼ cup shredded coconut in a small shallow dish. Scoop out about 1 tablespoon worth of the blended mixture and roll into a ball. Roll the ball in the shredded coconut flakes until fully coated, then place on a large parchment-lined dish. Repeat with the remaining mixture, which should make up to 12 to 14 energy bites depending on their size.

Place the energy bites in the freezer for at least 30 minutes to firm up, then enjoy. Transfer leftovers to a freezer-safe bag and store in the freezer for up to 3 months. Allow to thaw for 5 to 10 minutes before enjoying.

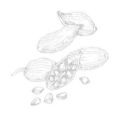

I adore these muffins… and they don't even have chocolate in them (and that's a pretty big deal)! Now, don't be alarmed when you see the word *aquafaba* in the ingredient list. This is our egg replacement, and it does an incredible job of keeping our muffins together. Yes, it is the liquid found in a can of chickpeas. But trust me, they don't make the muffins taste like chickpeas at all. If anything, they give impressive structure and lift to these beauties without making them get too heavy. Once you bake with it once, you will probably want to start baking with it more often. So save the liquid next time you drain a can of chickpeas and get ready to bake.

Cinnamon Swirl Banana Nut Muffins

MAKES 12 MUFFINS • PREP TIME: 20 MINUTES • COOKING TIME: 30 MINUTES

3 ripe bananas (300g)

⅓ cup (85g) plain unsweetened plant-based yogurt

⅓ cup (70g) packed light brown sugar

6 tablespoons aquafaba (the liquid from a can of chickpeas)

¼ cup avocado oil

1 tablespoon vanilla extract

1 tablespoon baking powder

½ teaspoon baking soda

½ teaspoon ground cinnamon

½ teaspoon kosher salt

2 cups (275g) all-purpose flour, spooned and leveled

⅓ cup (40g) chopped walnuts, plus ¼ cup (30g) for topping

4 tablespoons (52g) packed light brown sugar

1 teaspoon ground cinnamon

Turbinado sugar, for topping

Preheat the oven to 425°F, then line or grease a 12-cup muffin pan.

To a large bowl, add the bananas and, with a whisk or fork, mash them well. Add in the yogurt, brown sugar, aquafaba, oil, and vanilla, then whisk well until smooth.

Add the baking powder, baking soda, cinnamon, and salt, then whisk again until fully combined.

Pour in the flour, then with a spatula fold it into the batter until nice and smooth. Fold in the walnuts, then set aside.

Next, for the cinnamon swirl, mix the brown sugar and cinnamon together in a small bowl.

Add a 2 tablespoon scoop of batter to each muffin cup, then sprinkle a teaspoon of the cinnamon swirl mix on top. Divide and layer more batter on top to fill most of the cup then top each cup with a small sprinkle of coarse sugar and walnuts.

Once the pan is filled, place the muffins in the oven to bake for 5 minutes. While the muffins remain in the oven, reduce the temperature to 350°F and continue to bake the muffins for an additional 22 to 25 minutes.

Allow the muffins to cool in the pan for about 5 minutes, then transfer to a wire rack to continue cooling. Once fully cooled, the muffins can be stored for 2 to 3 days at room temperature in an airtight container or in the fridge for up to 1 week.

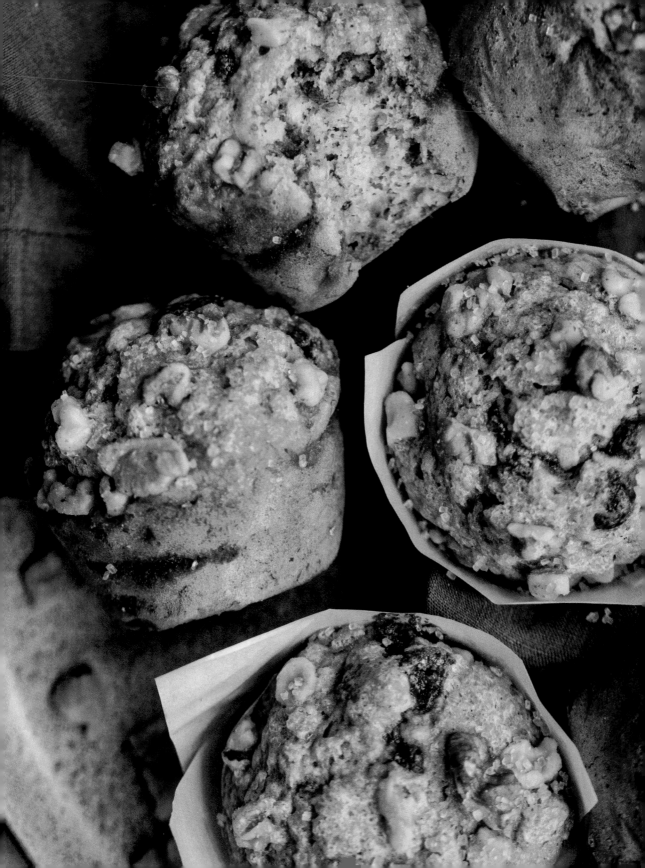

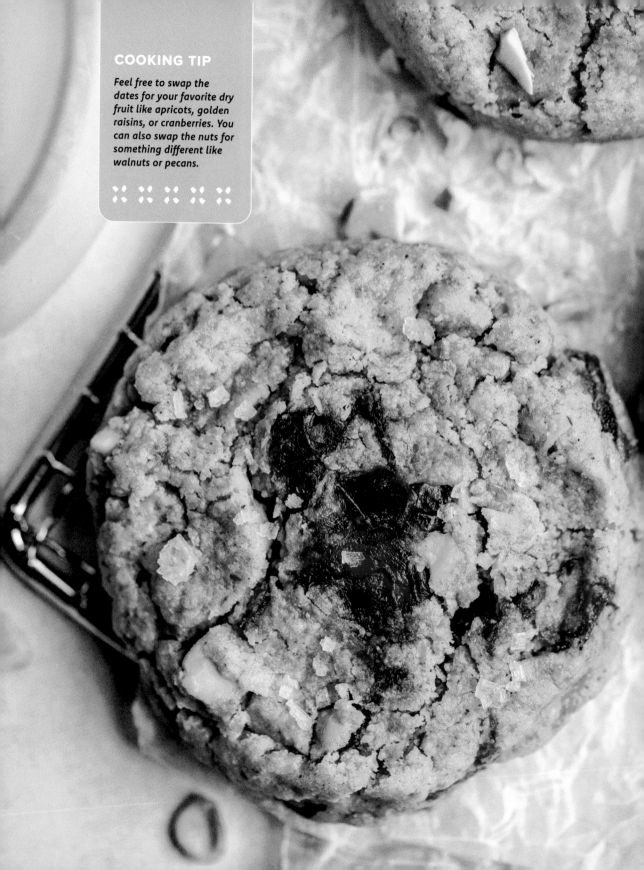

COOKING TIP

Feel free to swap the dates for your favorite dry fruit like apricots, golden raisins, or cranberries. You can also swap the nuts for something different like walnuts or pecans.

So when the hubby and I are relaxing after a long week of work, I can always count on him to turn to me and ask me to make a "treat." And when he says "treat," nine times out of ten that means he wants these cookies. This is a treat that also happens to pack in a bit of nutrition, and more important, satisfies our need for something sweet. So yes, you can have a gluten-free, high-fiber cookie that still manages to taste amazing. Now, while these are customizable, I must say that the pistachio and Medjool date combination is my current favorite. The dates add an extra bit of natural sweetness, which means we can also use less added sugar overall in this recipe. They are my miracle cookie.

Wholesome Date and Pistachio Cookies

MAKES 9 COOKIES • PREP TIME: 15 MINUTES • COOKING TIME: 11 MINUTES

2 tablespoons ground flaxseed

4 tablespoons almond milk

2/3 cup natural almond butter or peanut butter

1/3 cup maple syrup

3 tablespoons packed light brown sugar

1 teaspoon vanilla extract

1 teaspoon baking powder

1/2 teaspoon ground cinnamon

1/2 teaspoon ground cardamom

1/4 teaspoon kosher salt

1 cup rolled oats

1/3 cup pistachios, chopped

1/3 cup Medjool dates, pits removed and chopped

Preheat the oven to 350°F.

In a medium mixing bowl, combine the flaxseed and almond milk and whisk together. Allow to sit and gel for 5 minutes.

Add in the almond butter, maple syrup, brown sugar, vanilla, baking powder, cinnamon, cardamom, and salt, then whisk together until smooth.

To a mini food processor or blender, add 3/4 cup of the rolled oats and blend to make a flour. Add the flour and remaining 1/4 cup rolled oats, pistachios, and dates to the bowl with the almond butter mixture, then use a spatula to evenly mix it together.

Use a large cookie scoop to drop a scoop of cookie dough onto a parchment-lined baking sheet. Shape the dough into smooth balls, then use your palm to lightly flatten them.

Bake in the oven on the middle rack for about 11 minutes. If the cookies look slightly underdone, that's okay. They will continue to bake and properly set on the tray as they cool. Do not overbake or you will end up with a tough cookie.

Once out of the oven, take a spatula and very lightly press down on the cookies (this will give the same effect as dropping the tray on the counter to give you more of that perfect chewy center). Allow the cookies to completely cool before enjoying.

Okay, technically this makes two cookies. But that is what I personally consider a serving because one cookie is never enough. However, if you do stick to one cookie, then you will have another cookie to look forward to later.

Single-Serve Chocolate Chip Cookie

MAKES 2 COOKIES • PREP TIME: 10 MINUTES • COOKING TIME: 11 MINUTES

2 tablespoons natural almond butter or cashew butter

2 tablespoons packed light brown sugar

1 tablespoon granulated sugar

1 tablespoon plain unsweetened plant-based yogurt

Splash of vanilla extract

¼ teaspoon baking soda

Pinch of kosher salt

5 tablespoons (45g) all-purpose flour, spooned and leveled

2 to 3 tablespoons dairy-free chocolate chips or chunks

Preheat the oven to 350°F.

To a small mixing bowl, add the almond butter, brown sugar, and granulated sugar, then whisk together to fully combine.

Add the yogurt, vanilla, baking soda, and salt and stir well to evenly mix.

Fold in the flour until just combined, then stir in the chocolate chips. Avoid overmixing the dough. Place the dough in the freezer for 10 to 15 minutes to firm up.

Divide the dough into two equal-size dough balls. Place them on a parchment-lined baking sheet and slightly press down on the dough balls to flatten slightly, then push in a few extra pieces of chocolate chips on top.

Bake for 11 to 12 minutes or until the edges appear lightly golden. Smack the tray down on your kitchen counter to help flatten the cookies a little. Allow to cool on the baking sheet for at least 10 minutes to firm up further before enjoying.

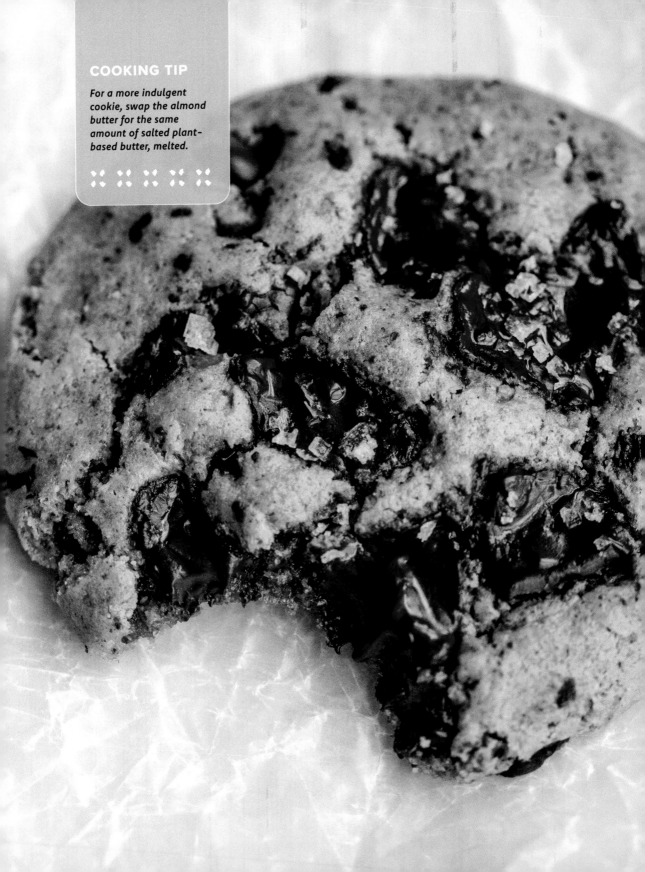

COOKING TIP

For a more indulgent
cookie, swap the almond
butter for the same
amount of salted plant-
based butter, melted.

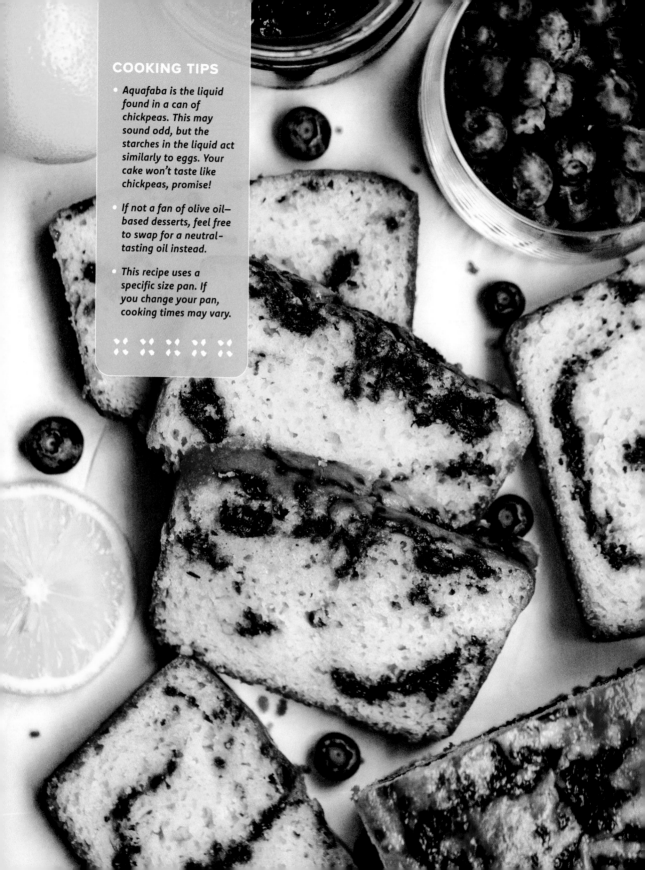

COOKING TIPS

- *Aquafaba is the liquid found in a can of chickpeas. This may sound odd, but the starches in the liquid act similarly to eggs. Your cake won't taste like chickpeas, promise!*

- *If not a fan of olive oil—based desserts, feel free to swap for a neutral-tasting oil instead.*

- *This recipe uses a specific size pan. If you change your pan, cooking times may vary.*

Lemon and blueberry are such an iconic duo, and while yes, the classic lemon blueberry loaf does exist and is fantastic, I raise you a blueberry jam swirl in each slice instead. This cake is delicate and moist with just enough sweetness to satisfy and a lot of emphasis on getting the most flavor out of our ingredients. So to emphasize those sweet lemony notes, I rubbed the sugar with the lemon zest at the very start to help infuse more of the natural lemony oils into the loaf. It makes the biggest difference in flavor and further helps enhance the taste of the blueberries from the jam (bonus points if you make your own). Then it's a matter of mixing your batter together in one bowl, filling your loaf pan, swirling in your jam, and baking. Cut into it, marvel at the swirls, then enjoy it very much like I did.

Lemon Blueberry Swirl Loaf

SERVES 8 • PREP TIME: 15 MINUTES • COOKING TIME: 50 MINUTES

¾ cup (160g) granulated sugar

Zest and juice of 2 lemons

¼ cup unsweetened soy milk

¼ cup aquafaba (the liquid from a can of chickpeas)

¼ cup extra-virgin olive oil or avocado oil

¼ cup (75g) plain unsweetened plant-based yogurt

1 tablespoon vanilla extract

1 tablespoon baking powder

½ teaspoon baking soda

½ teaspoon kosher salt

2 cups cup all-purpose flour, spooned and leveled

8 tablespoons store-bought blueberry jam or homemade Lemon Blueberry Chia Jam (page 224)

Preheat the oven to 375°F. Line an 8 × 4 × 2 ½-inch nonstick loaf pan with parchment paper and set to the side.

To a large mixing bowl, add the sugar and lemon zest. Rub the sugar between your fingers to help release the natural oils in the zest.

Into a large measuring cup, add ¼ cup of the lemon juice, then add the soy milk. Whisk together and set aside.

To the bowl with the sugar and zest, add the aquafaba, oil, yogurt, and vanilla, then whisk to fully combine.

At this point, pour in the milk mixture, then add the baking powder, baking soda, and salt and whisk again.

Add the flour, then slowly start to whisk the flour into the batter. Once mostly combined, switch your whisk to a spatula and continue to fold the flour into the batter until smooth.

Add the jam to a small bowl along with 2 tablespoons warm water and stir well to loosen it up.

Pour half the batter into the loaf pan, then dollop 6 generous tablespoons of blueberry jam along the length of the loaf. Use a butter knife to swirl the jam into the batter. I like to do a few figure eight motions or go back and forth in the batter. Pour the remaining batter overtop, then add the remaining jam along the length of the loaf and again swirl the jam into the batter.

Bake the loaf in the oven for 50 to 60 minutes or until a toothpick comes out clean. Allow the loaf to cool for 15 minutes in its pan, then transfer to a wire cooling rack to continue cooling. Slice, then enjoy.

I can sense your trepidation, but stay with me. Before you scoff at the idea of chickpeas in a dessert, just hear me out. I've been making "cookie dough" using chickpeas for a very long time as a dietitian. When I first saw the recipe my dietitian group was sharing for us to use during kids' events, I was convinced it would flop hard. But to my surprise, the kids were all about this plant-based riff on classic cookie dough. It still is one of my most popular food demos for kids. I have modified the recipe a lot over the years. This is probably my favorite version, in delicious chocolate bar form. And even still, I'm shocked at how good they are.

Chickpea Cookie Dough Bars

MAKES 8 BARS • PREP TIME: 30 MINUTES

1 15-ounce can chickpeas, drained and rinsed

1 teaspoon baking soda

2 cups boiling water, plus more as needed

⅓ cup natural almond butter or peanut butter

½ cup oat flour, spooned and leveled

3 tablespoons maple syrup

4 tablespoons packed light brown sugar

1 teaspoon vanilla extract

½ teaspoon kosher salt

⅓ cup vegan mini chocolate chips

1 4-ounce bar vegan dark chocolate

Flaky sea salt, for sprinkling

Line an 8 × 4 × 2 ½-inch loaf pan with parchment paper and set aside.

Place the chickpeas in a large heat-safe bowl. Add the baking soda and add enough boiling water to cover the chickpeas. Give the chickpeas a mix and allow to sit for 15 minutes.

Drain and rinse the chickpeas, then fill the bowl with cold water. Rub the chickpeas between your fingers to release the skins. The skins should float to the top. Scoop them out to discard, then drain the chickpeas well.

To a food processor, add the chickpeas, almond butter, flour, maple syrup, brown sugar, vanilla, and salt. Run the food processor to blend the ingredients together, scraping down the sides as needed until you have a uniform sticky dough ball form. Remove the blade of the food processor, then stir in the chocolate chips.

Transfer the dough to the prepared loaf pan, and using a spatula, press the dough down and spread it out evenly across the pan. Make sure that it is pressed all the way into the corners. Smooth the top out, then place the pan in the freezer for up to 30 minutes.

Break up your chocolate bar in a small microwave-safe bowl, and microwave on high for 30 seconds. Use a spatula to mix some of the melted chocolate. Place the bowl back in the microwave for 15 seconds, then stir and repeat in intervals until most of the chocolate has melted. Continue to stir until the remaining chocolate has fully melted.

Pour the chocolate over the cookie dough, and quickly spread it to cover completely. Sprinkle the top with flaky sea salt, then place the pan in the fridge for 5 minutes to fully set and harden.

Run a sharp knife under hot water for a minute. Use it to cut the chocolate-coated dough into 8 equal bars. Enjoy and store leftovers in the freezer for up to 2 months.

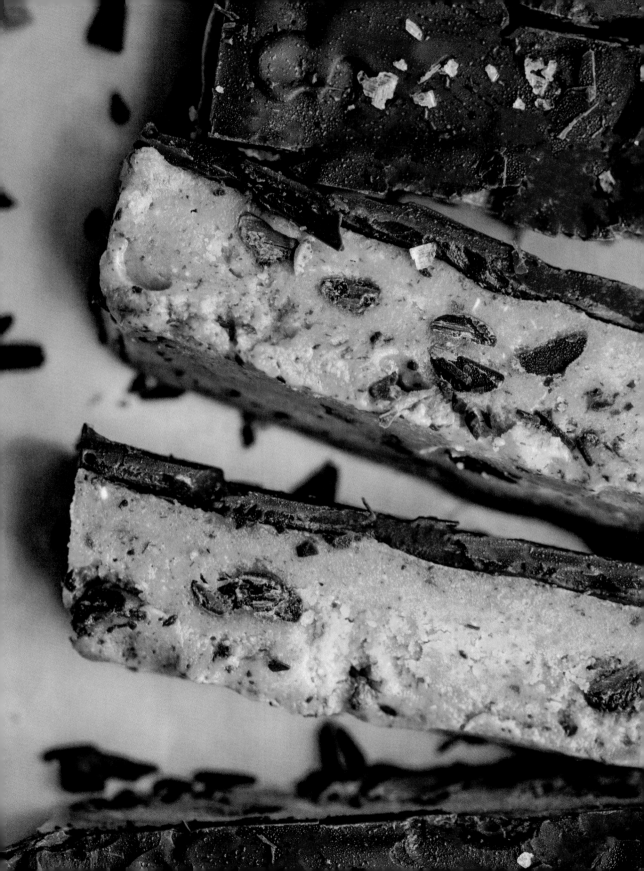

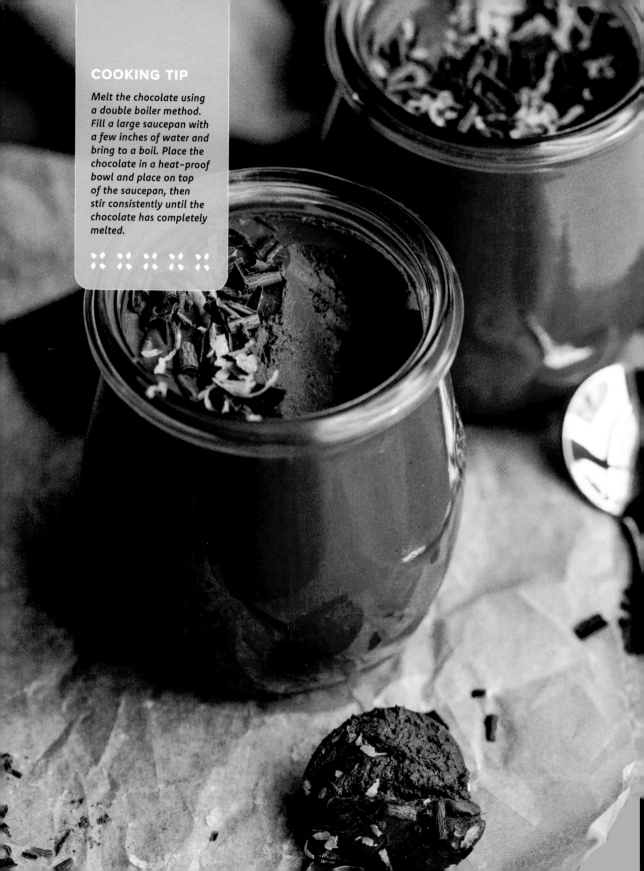

COOKING TIP

Melt the chocolate using a double boiler method. Fill a large saucepan with a few inches of water and bring to a boil. Place the chocolate in a heat-proof bowl and place on top of the saucepan, then stir consistently until the chocolate has completely melted.

Chocolate and lemon don't seem to be a pair that should go together, but let me show you why it is one of my new favorite combos. I probably wouldn't have even tried this pairing if it wasn't for a little shop I stumbled upon in San Diego called Nibble Chocolate. They had a variety of chocolate truffles in different flavors, and the one I thought I would like least was the one I ended up loving the most. The bright citrusy notes of the lemon balanced out the rich and earthy flavors of the chocolate. So when I was thinking about this mousse, all I could think about was adding those bright lemony notes to it. And it truly did not disappoint.

Chocolate Lemon Mousse

SERVES 6 • PREP TIME: 15 MINUTES • COOKING TIME: 3 MINUTES

5 ounces 70% dark chocolate bars

12 ounces (340g) silken tofu, brought to room temperature

3 tablespoons maple syrup

2 tablespoons unsweetened Dutch-processed cocoa powder

1 teaspoon espresso powder

Zest of 1 lemon, plus more for topping

½ teaspoon kosher salt

Flaky sea salt, for sprinkling

Start by melting the chocolate. To melt the chocolate in the microwave, break the chocolate bars into smaller pieces in a small microwave-safe bowl. Place in the microwave for 30 seconds, then stir. Microwave the chocolate in 15-second intervals, stirring each time until the chocolate is fully melted (for me this took 3 15-second intervals).

Place the tofu, maple syrup, cocoa powder, espresso powder, lemon zest, and kosher salt into a high-speed blender or food processor. Blend the mixture until completely smooth, scraping down the sides as needed.

Pour in all the melted chocolate and continue to blend until completely smooth, scraping down the sides as needed.

Divide the mousse between 6 small dessert glasses. Place the mousse in the fridge for at least 30 minutes to firm up. If making ahead, place the mousse in small airtight jars and store in the fridge for up to 3 days. To serve, allow the mousse to sit out at room temperature for a few minutes, then top with extra lemon zest and a sprinkle of flaky salt, then enjoy.

Onigiri are Japanese rice balls that are made using steamed rice that is compressed. When pressed together, rice can be shaped into balls, triangles, or even cylinders, then wrapped with a piece of nori. Adding some shredded seasoned tofu to onigiri adds protein, extra iron, and calcium. Not to mention, its compact size also makes it a fun way to eat rice on the go.

High-Protein Onigiri

SERVES 6 • PREP TIME: 15 MINUTES • COOKING TIME: 25 MINUTES

1½ cups sushi rice or medium-grain white rice, rinsed

8 ounces (about ½ a package) super-firm high-protein tofu (see page 122)

½ tablespoon cornstarch

1 tablespoon gochujang

½ tablespoon tamari

½ tablespoon avocado oil

½ tablespoon rice vinegar

Kosher salt to taste (optional)

1 sheet of nori (optional)

Preheat the oven to 425°F. Line a baking sheet with parchment paper.

Add your rinsed rice to a large saucepan or rice cooker and cook according to package instructions. Once cooked, remove the rice from the heat and allow to stand covered for 10 minutes, then fluff with a fork.

Place a box grater over the prepared baking sheet and grate the tofu over the largest holes of the grater. Sprinkle the tofu with the cornstarch and toss to coat.

In a small bowl, add the gochujang, tamari, oil, and vinegar, then whisk together until smooth. Pour it over the tofu, then toss together until evenly coated.

Spread the tofu out on the prepared baking sheet, then bake in the oven for 12 minutes. Give the tofu a toss, then bake for another 5 to 8 minutes.

When the rice is warm and safe to touch with your hands, add the tofu, then stir well to combine.

You can shape your onigiri in different ways by using your hands or with an onigiri mold. If using a mold, spray the mold with water and add a sprinkle of salt. Fill the mold with the rice, press the shape together, then release the onigiri from the mold. Alternatively, place a piece of plastic wrap on a smooth surface and add a scoop of about ⅓ cup rice to it. Sprinkle the rice with salt, then gather the corners of the plastic wrap together and twist to help compact the rice. Use your hands to firmly form the rice into a triangular shape, making sure it is holding its shape. You can repeat this process using the same piece of plastic wrap.

Remove the onigiri from the plastic wrap to enjoy or wrap with a strip of nori, if desired. To do this, cut your sheet of nori in half, then cut each half into 5 thin strips widthwise. Stand the onigiri on the middle of a strip of nori, then fold the ends up to touch the center of the onigiri from the front and back. Serve and enjoy!

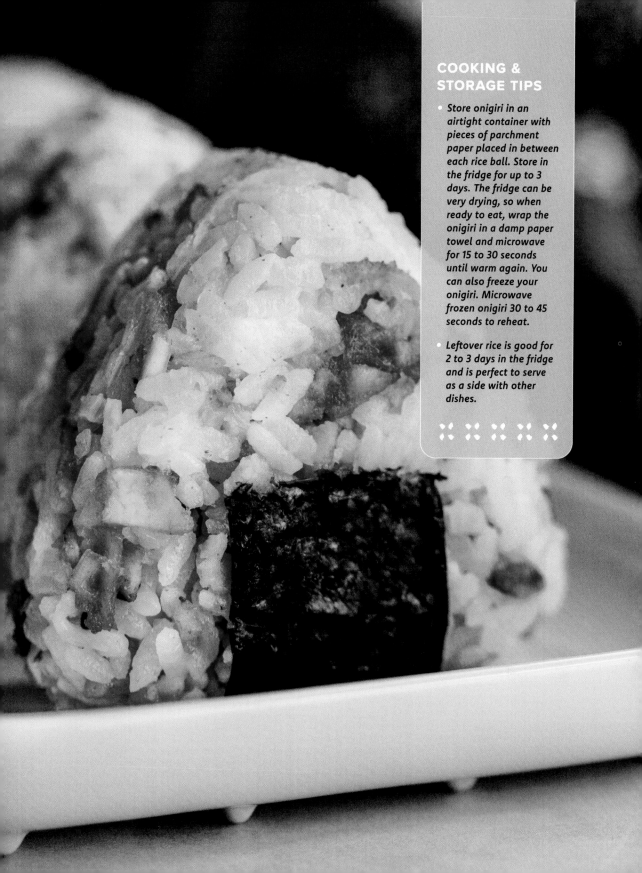

COOKING & STORAGE TIPS

- Store onigiri in an airtight container with pieces of parchment paper placed in between each rice ball. Store in the fridge for up to 3 days. The fridge can be very drying, so when ready to eat, wrap the onigiri in a damp paper towel and microwave for 15 to 30 seconds until warm again. You can also freeze your onigiri. Microwave frozen onigiri 30 to 45 seconds to reheat.

- Leftover rice is good for 2 to 3 days in the fridge and is perfect to serve as a side with other dishes.

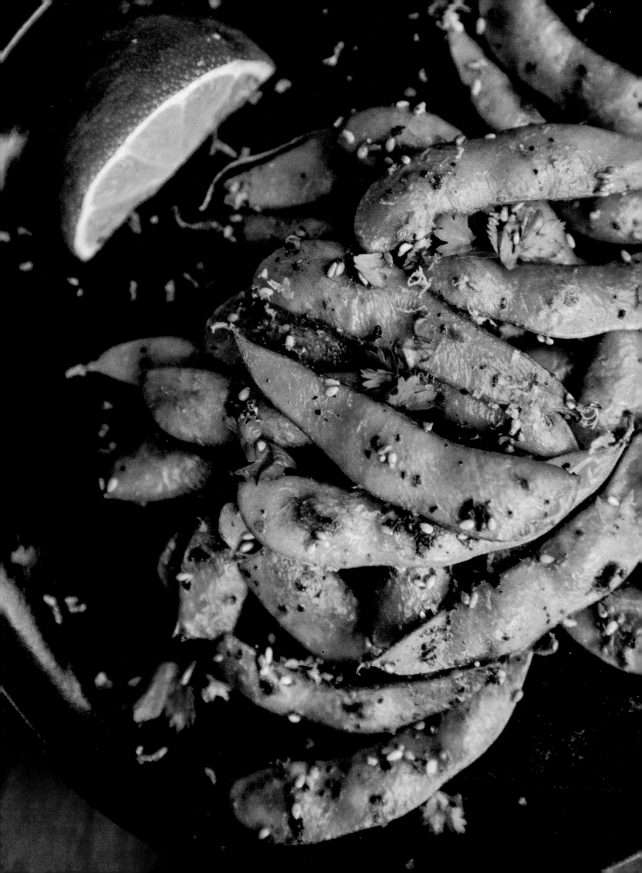

I'm content just eating plain edamame with a little salt as a snack. I've been obsessed with it ever since I was served my first bowl at my first sushi restaurant. My friends explained to me how you were supposed to eat it from the pod, and it didn't take long for me to demolish that whole bowl. Fast forward to today, I still love to snack on edamame, especially since it's a great source of plant-based protein. However, I became even more of a fan of this snack when I started flavoring it beyond just adding salt. Just a little citrus, sesame oil, and spice can take your edamame experience to a whole new level. This is the snack I now love to grab when I'm watching my favorite shows.

Blistered Sesame Lime Edamame

SERVES 4 • PREP TIME: 5 MINUTES • COOKING TIME: 6 MINUTES

1 10-ounce bag frozen edamame in pods

2 teaspoons toasted sesame oil

1 tablespoon sesame seeds

½ teaspoon garlic powder

½ teaspoon gochugaru or chili powder

1 teaspoon maple syrup

Zest of 1 lime

Juice of ½ lime

Kosher salt to taste

Heat a large nonstick skillet over medium-low heat. Once hot, add the frozen edamame to the pan and spread the pods out evenly into a single layer.

Allow the pods to cook undisturbed for 2 to 3 minutes to sear. Give the edamame a toss and spread them out again over the pan and cook again for an additional 2 to 3 minutes or until you see some light browning on the surface of your pods.

Lower the heat to the lowest setting, then add the sesame oil, sesame seeds, garlic powder, and gochugaru and stir well to coat for about 1 minute until the garlic is fragrant.

Add the maple syrup, lime zest, and juice as well as a pinch of salt and toss again to evenly coat the edamame. Adjust the salt to taste and serve.

Whenever I go home to visit my mom, I can usually count on her making me *plátanos fritos* (fried green plantains). She knows how much I love them, and I know what a labor of love they are, so each time is special. Traditionally, this is fried, but in an effort to find a less messy and oil-splashing solution, I turned to my air fryer. It took some experimenting, but I found a way to make some really good-looking plátanos "fritos" using this method. And they taste as close to home as I can get.

Air-Fried Plantains

SERVES 4 • PREP TIME: 15 MINUTES • COOKING TIME: 15 MINUTES

2 green unripe plantains

2 to 3 tablespoons avocado oil or favorite high-heat oil, plus more as needed

Kosher salt to taste

Mashed avocado or Everything Sauce (page 220), for serving

With a knife, cut the ends of the plantains, then carefully peel off the skin. Cut the plantains into 1-inch pieces, then place in a medium mixing bowl with 1 tablespoon of the oil and toss to coat completely, add more oil if needed.

Place the plantains in an air fryer, making sure the pieces are not piled on top of one another, then bake for 10 minutes at 320° to 325°F.

Transfer the plantains into the same mixing bowl. While the plantains are warm, flatten them into ¼-inch-thick coins. To flatten the plantains, you can use a tostonera or place the plantain pieces between two pieces of parchment paper, then press down using a flat-bottomed mug.

Add the flattened plantains back to the bowl, then coat completely with the remaining oil. If not fully coated, use an additional drizzle of oil.

Place back in the air fryer at 320° to 325°F and cook for an additional 5 to 7 minutes until nice and golden. Serve immediately with a pinch of salt and some mashed avocado.

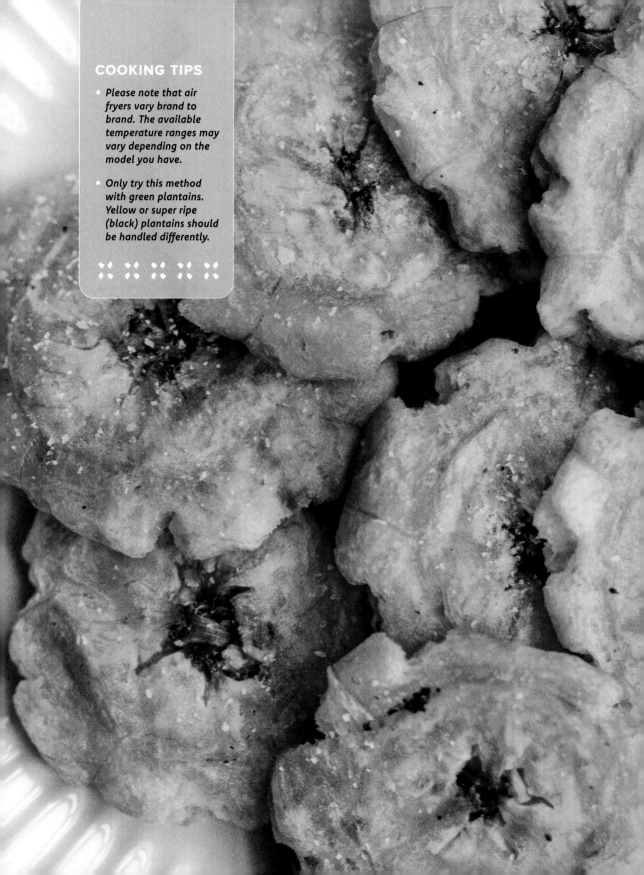

COOKING TIPS

- *Please note that air fryers vary brand to brand. The available temperature ranges may vary depending on the model you have.*

- *Only try this method with green plantains. Yellow or super ripe (black) plantains should be handled differently.*

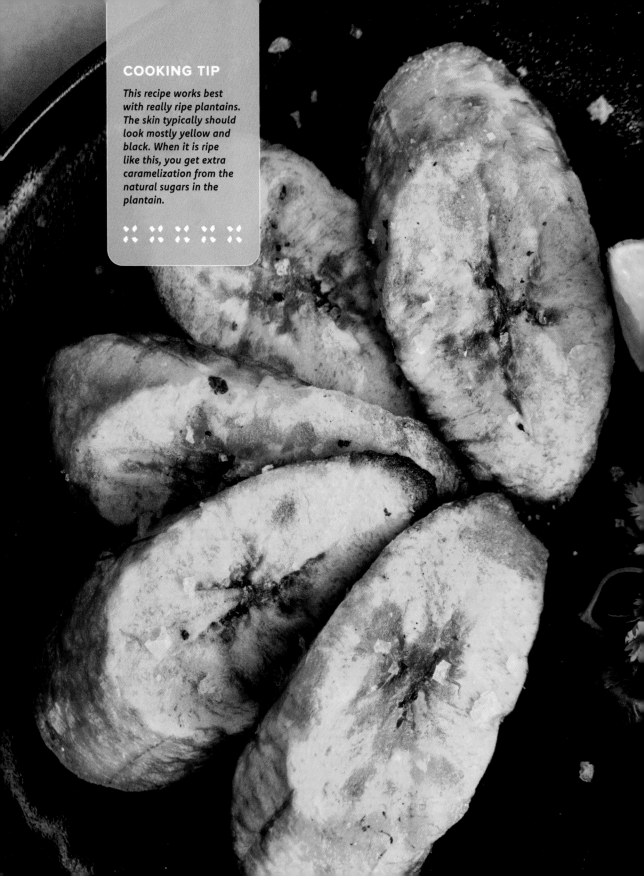

COOKING TIP

This recipe works best with really ripe plantains. The skin typically should look mostly yellow and black. When it is ripe like this, you get extra caramelization from the natural sugars in the plantain.

Plantains can also be baked sweet. They are typically referred to as *maduros*. They make a fantastic addition to savory bowls for a little play on savory-sweet, but I've grown up eating them on their own, too. Typically, my mom would either make fried savory plantains or sweet plantains depending on what she picked up at the store. I could never decide which I liked better, so I always requested both when they were available. So, of course, I had to give you both savory and sweet preparations.

Baked Plátanos Maduros

SERVES 4 • PREP TIME: 10 MINUTES • COOKING TIME: 20 MINUTES

2 ripe plantains, peeled and sliced into ½-inch-thick slices

2 tablespoons avocado oil or high-heat avocado oil spray

Kosher salt to taste

Preheat the oven to 425°F.

Place the plantains on a parchment-lined baking sheet and brush or spray both sides with oil. Place the plantains in the oven to cook for 15 minutes, then flip and roast for another 5 to 10 minutes until golden.

Sprinkle the plantains with a little salt when they come out of the oven, then enjoy.

Roasting chickpeas is fun, but you can roast other beans, too. Personally, my second favorite beans to roast are butter beans. These big beans are a fun snack, especially when seasoned well. For the flavor, I used some Old Bay seasoning. For the crisp, I coated the beans in some nutritional yeast and potato starch. Then, just let them get crispy in the oven using a double-bake method. The best protein- and fiber-packed snack!

Crispy Old Bay Beans

SERVES 3 TO 4 • PREP TIME: 5 MINUTES • COOKING TIME: 30 MINUTES

1 15-ounce can butter beans, drained and rinsed

1 tablespoon potato starch

1 tablespoon nutritional yeast

1 teaspoon Old Bay seasoning

½ teaspoon dried thyme

½ teaspoon ground coriander

Kosher salt to taste

1 tablespoon avocado oil, plus more as needed

Jalapeño Lime Crema (optional, page 219)

Preheat your oven to 400°F.

Place your drained beans on a clean kitchen towel and gently pat dry.

Transfer the beans to a medium mixing bowl with the potato starch, nutritional yeast, Old Bay, thyme, coriander, and a pinch of salt. Drizzle the oil over top and toss again to coat, using more oil if needed.

Spread the beans out in a single layer on a parchment-lined baking sheet. Bake in the oven on the middle rack for 20 minutes. Remove from the oven and allow the beans to cool for 10 minutes.

Give the beans a toss and place them back in the oven for 5 to 8 minutes to give them a final crisp. Serve as is or enjoy with some Jalapeño Lime Crema as a dip.

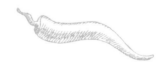

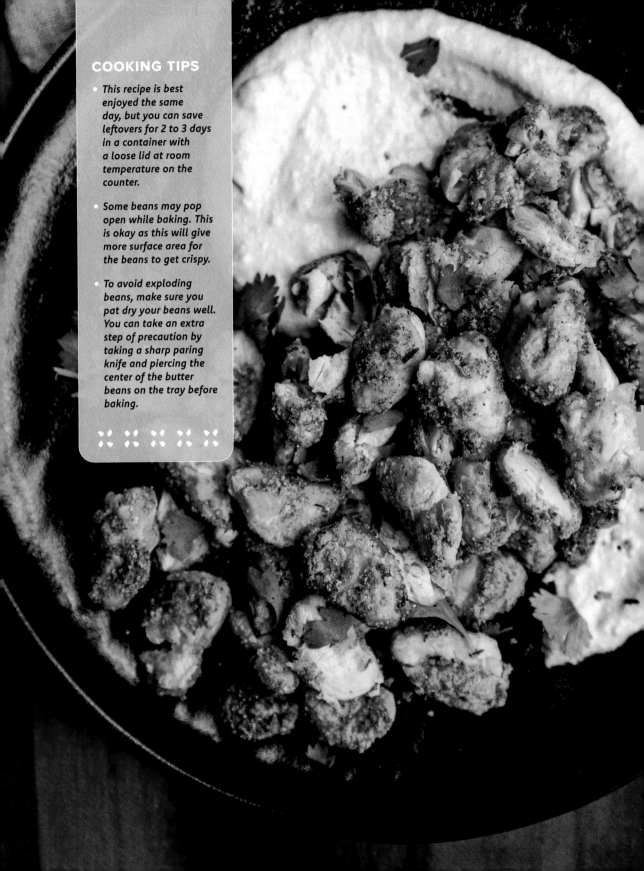

COOKING TIPS

- This recipe is best enjoyed the same day, but you can save leftovers for 2 to 3 days in a container with a loose lid at room temperature on the counter.

- Some beans may pop open while baking. This is okay as this will give more surface area for the beans to get crispy.

- To avoid exploding beans, make sure you pat dry your beans well. You can take an extra step of precaution by taking a sharp paring knife and piercing the center of the butter beans on the tray before baking.

CHAPTER 8

I stand by the fact that if you have one to two REALLY GOOD SAUCES in your fridge, you can build incredible meals with MINIMAL EFFORT. So here is a chapter with plenty of sauces and other condiments to keep your MEALS INTERESTING and your bellies happy.

Sauceology

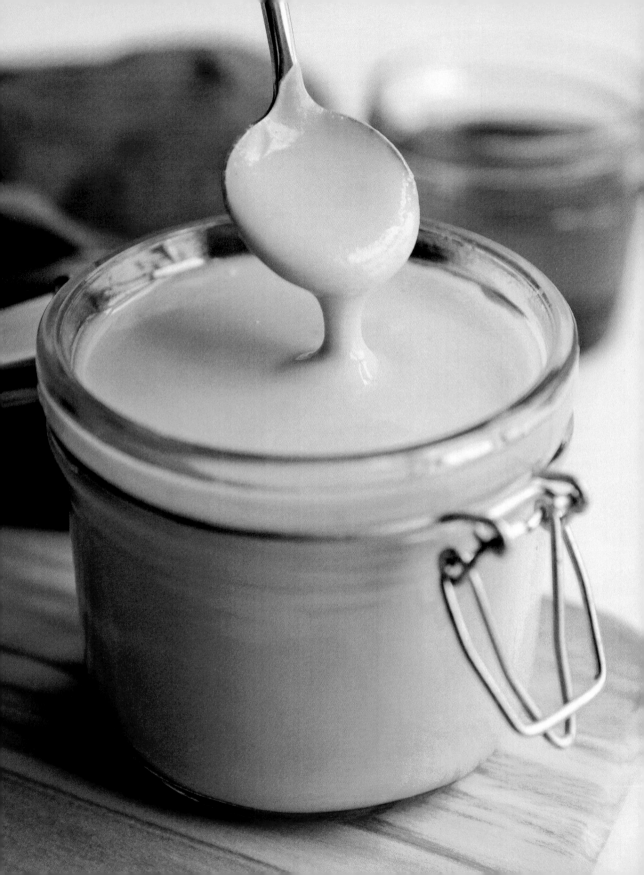

This has been a go-to sauce for years and emulates one of my favorite condiments of all time, honey mustard. To make this plant-based we are using maple syrup instead of honey. And, to make it the perfect creamy consistency, stirring in some plant-based yogurt. It comes together in minutes and is ready to use to add some sweet, tangy flavor to your favorite bowls or other dishes.

Maple Dijon Dressing

MAKES ABOUT ½ CUP DRESSING • PREP TIME: 5 MINUTES

2 tablespoons Dijon mustard, plus more as needed

2 tablespoons maple syrup, plus more as needed

3 tablespoons plain unsweetened plant-based yogurt, plus more as needed

1 small garlic clove, grated

2 teaspoons lemon juice (about a small wedge of lemon)

Kosher salt to taste

Combine the mustard, maple syrup, yogurt, garlic, lemon juice, and a pinch of salt together in a small bowl. Whisk together until fully combined and smooth, then taste and adjust ingredient amounts based on preference (more mustard if you need more tang, etc.). Use this dressing to drizzle over your favorite bowls or salads or use as a dip.

Pico de gallo has been a steady condiment for a good portion of my life. At its core, it is incredibly simple, using a base of tomatoes, onion, pepper, cilantro, and lime. I would prep this all the time and use as a way to quickly add some freshness and zingy flavor to a meal. In making it regularly, I have created many variations of this classic Mexican condiment, and this is probably my favorite version. It emphasizes the bold citrus flavors and brings an element of creaminess with the addition of avocado that makes it ultra satisfying.

Avocado Pico de Gallo

MAKES 1 ½ CUPS • PREP TIME: 10 MINUTES

2 plum tomatoes, diced

¼ medium white onion, finely diced

1 to 2 serrano peppers, stems removed, minced

⅓ cup fresh cilantro leaves, minced

Zest and juice of 1 lime

½ teaspoon kosher salt, plus more to taste

1 medium avocado, cubed

To a medium mixing bowl, add the tomatoes, onion, peppers, cilantro, lime zest and juice, and salt.

Stir the mixture well, taste, and adjust the salt to your liking.

Right before serving, carefully fold in the avocado with a spatula to prevent it from getting mushy. Serve as a topping in tacos and bowls or serve with chips.

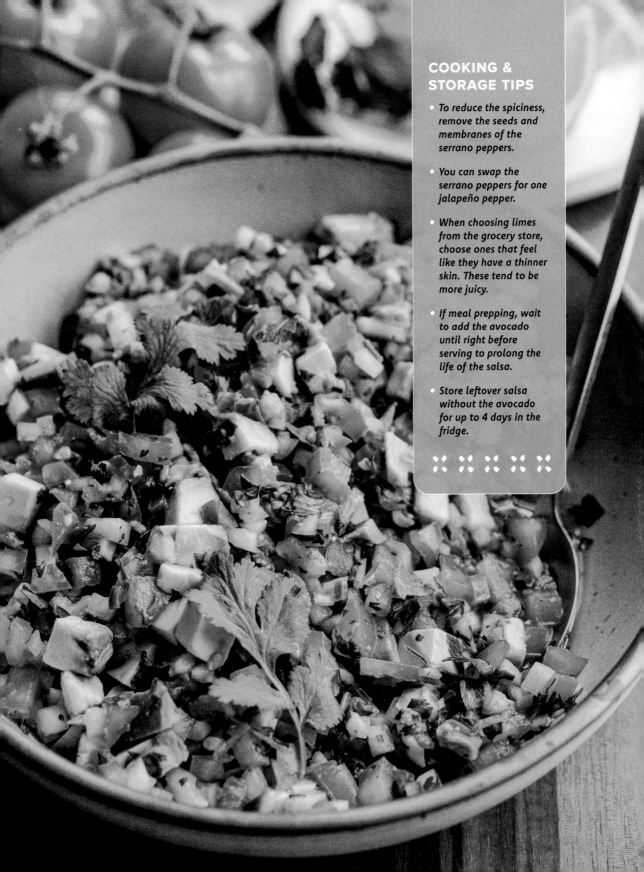

COOKING & STORAGE TIPS

- *To reduce the spiciness, remove the seeds and membranes of the serrano peppers.*

- *You can swap the serrano peppers for one jalapeño pepper.*

- *When choosing limes from the grocery store, choose ones that feel like they have a thinner skin. These tend to be more juicy.*

- *If meal prepping, wait to add the avocado until right before serving to prolong the life of the salsa.*

- *Store leftover salsa without the avocado for up to 4 days in the fridge.*

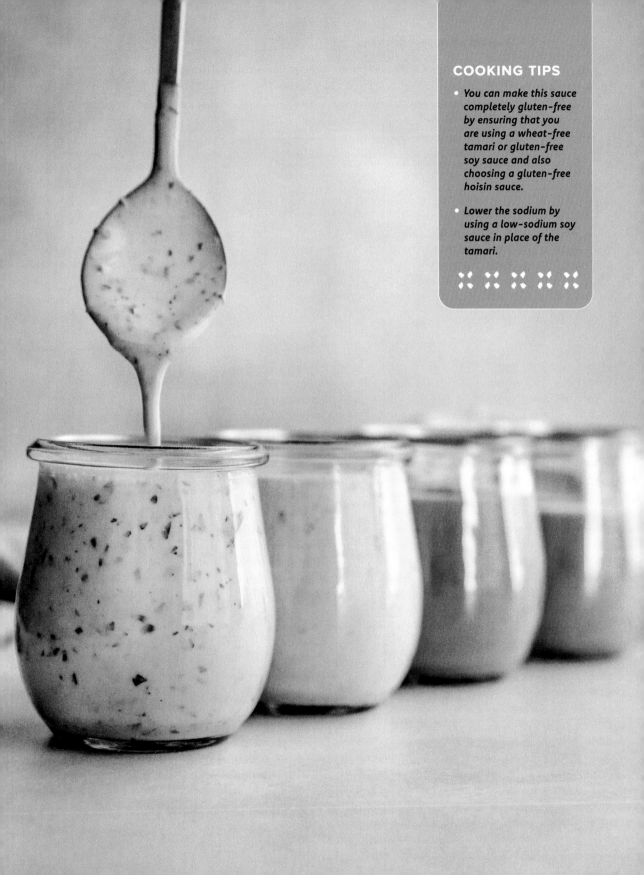

COOKING TIPS

- *You can make this sauce completely gluten-free by ensuring that you are using a wheat-free tamari or gluten-free soy sauce and also choosing a gluten-free hoisin sauce.*

- *Lower the sodium by using a low-sodium soy sauce in place of the tamari.*

I rely a lot on tahini sauces, and when you whisk a good-quality tahini with the right ingredients, you can build sauces that can complete a meal and really take it to the next level. To best showcase how versatile this simple whole food ingredient is, I've compiled a list of my absolute favorites.

Tahini Sauces

Sweet Tahini Hoisin Sauce

MAKES ¾ CUP • PREP TIME: 5 MINUTES

I am all about creamy sauces, and this one is good enough to drink. Tahini helps give this sauce a nice velvety texture while still providing a great deal of nutritional benefit. Using whole fats like tahini helps provide monounsaturated fatty acids that are good for your heart. You also get fiber and antioxidants with each delicious spoonful.

¼ cup good-quality tahini (see page 59)

2 tablespoons hoisin sauce

2 tablespoons maple syrup

1 tablespoon tamari

1 tablespoon rice vinegar

1 teaspoon garlic powder

Combine the tahini, hoisin sauce, maple syrup, tamari, vinegar, and garlic powder in a small bowl and whisk until smooth. As you whisk, you should notice the tahini sauce getting thicker in consistency.

Add 3 tablespoons water and whisk again. If the sauce is too thick, whisk in 1 tablespoon of water at a time until the sauce is at your desired consistency.

Store leftover sauce in an airtight container and place in the fridge for up to 7 days. Allow the sauce to come back to room temperature before using.

Creamy Caesar Tahini Dressing

MAKES ABOUT 1 CUP • PREP TIME: 10 MINUTES

Of all the tahini sauces I make, this is the one I use most often. The tahini in this makes for the perfect creamy base, and its earthy tones help bring out more of the tangy and umami-packed flavors. It's great for a classic Caesar salad but also a perfect dip for vegetables, too.

⅓ cup good-quality tahini (see page 59)

1 garlic clove, crushed or grated

Zest and juice of ½ lemon

2 teaspoons capers, finely minced

2 tablespoons caper brine from a caper jar

1 teaspoon Dijon mustard

1 teaspoon yellow or white miso paste

3 tablespoons nutritional yeast

Kosher salt and freshly ground black pepper to taste

In a medium mixing bowl, combine the tahini, garlic, lemon zest and juice, capers, caper brine, mustard, miso paste, nutritional yeast, and a pinch of salt and pepper, then whisk.

As the mixture thickens, pour in ⅓ cup cold water and whisk until creamy and smooth. If the dressing is too thick, add additional water 1 tablespoon at a time until the dressing is at your desired consistency.

Taste and adjust salt and pepper as desired.

Orange Ginger Tahini Dressing

MAKES ABOUT ¾ CUP • PREP TIME: 5 MINUTES

Creamy, bright, and zingy. I love the taste of orange and ginger together, and when blended into this tahini sauce it becomes pure magic.

4 tablespoons good-quality tahini (see page 59), plus more as needed

1 garlic clove, grated

1 teaspoon grated fresh ginger

1 teaspoon orange zest

4 tablespoons orange juice

1 tablespoon tamari

1 tablespoon maple syrup

2 teaspoons rice vinegar

Kosher salt to taste

To a small jar or bowl, add the tahini, garlic, ginger, orange zest, orange juice, tamari, maple syrup, vinegar, and a pinch of salt, then whisk until smooth.

As you whisk, your sauce will thicken. If the sauce is too thick, add 1 tablespoon of cold water at a time while whisking until you achieve your desired consistency. If your sauce becomes accidentally too thin, whisk in 1 tablespoon of tahini. Adjust salt to taste, then enjoy over salads and your favorite nourishing bowls.

 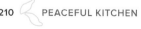

Roasted Garlic and Herb Tahini Dressing

MAKES ABOUT 2/3 CUP • PREP TIME: **10 MINUTES** • COOK TIME: **30 MINUTES**

Can a dressing bring you joy? I believe it absolutely can. That joy comes in the form of roasting garlic until it's nice and jammy, then mixing it with tahini to make a dressing that I love to pour on everything and anything. I especially love to make a big batch of this at the start of the week and can confirm that it makes me more likely to eat and enjoy my veggies that much more.

1 small garlic head (about 8 garlic cloves)

2 teaspoons extra-virgin olive oil

1/3 cup good-quality tahini (see page 59)

2 tablespoons plain unsweetened plant-based yogurt

Zest and juice of 1 lemon

1 teaspoon Dijon mustard

1 tablespoon maple syrup

1/4 teaspoon kosher salt, plus more as needed

Pinch of freshly ground black pepper

3 tablespoons minced cilantro or parsley

Heat the oven to 400°F.

Using a sharp knife, cut 1/4 inch to 1/2 inch off the top of the garlic bulb to expose the cloves. Place the bulb on a piece of foil that can wrap the bulb completely, then drizzle the exposed cloves with the oil. Wrap the garlic in the foil, then place the bulb on a baking sheet and place in the oven for 30 to 40 minutes until the cloves are completely soft and caramelized.

When the bulb is safe to handle, squeeze the garlic cloves out onto a cutting board. Smash the cloves with the flat side of your knife to make a paste, then scrape it up and place in a small bowl.

Add the tahini, yogurt, lemon zest and juice, mustard, maple syrup, salt, and pepper, then whisk to combine. As you whisk, your mixture will start to thicken. Start by adding 4 tablespoons water and whisk again until smooth. If still too thick, add water 1 tablespoon at a time, while whisking, until you achieve your desired creamy consistency, then fold in the herbs until well incorporated.

Store this dressing in an airtight container in the fridge for up to 7 days. This can be used to top salads and nourishing bowls or even to dress up your favorite veggies.

Pesto is an incredible condiment that can save you so much time during the workweek. Just prep it in advance and you can use it to instantly flavor any meal of your choosing. Toss it with vegetables, use it as a spread in sandwiches, or make some easy pasta or Charred Scallion Pesto Baked Gnocchi (page 144) with it.

Now, there are two special things about this sauce. First, we are adding some smoky notes of charred scallion and garlic for extra umami flavor. Second, we are giving it a boost of protein by using some pepitas, hemp hearts, and nutritional yeast. And even with these modifications, it still manages to pack in all of those familiar flavors with a little bit of something new to excite your taste buds.

Charred Scallion Pesto

MAKES 1 CUP • PREP TIME: 15 MINUTES • COOK TIME: 7 MINUTES

3 scallions

3 garlic cloves, smashed

1½ cups packed fresh basil, stems removed

3 tablespoons pepitas

2 tablespoons hemp hearts

3 tablespoons nutritional yeast

Zest and juice of 1 large lemon

¼ teaspoon kosher salt, plus more to taste

⅓ cup extra-virgin olive oil

Place a heavy-botttomed skillet over medium heat. Once hot, add the scallions and press them down into the surface of the pan with a spatula. Sear the scallions for 2 to 3 minutes, then flip and sear again for 2 to 3 minutes or until nicely charred. Add in the garlic and char for 1 minute on each side.

Transfer the scallions to a cutting board. Discard the root then roughly chop the scallions into pieces.

To a food processor, add the scallions, garlic, basil, pepitas, hemp hearts, nutritional yeast, lemon zest and juice, and salt. Pulse the mixture together until a paste begins to form, scraping the sides down as needed.

While the food processor is running, slowly stream in the oil to create a sauce. Continue to blend and scrape down the sides as needed until you get a thick, mostly smooth sauce. Adjust salt to taste, then store in an airtight container in the fridge for up to 5 days.

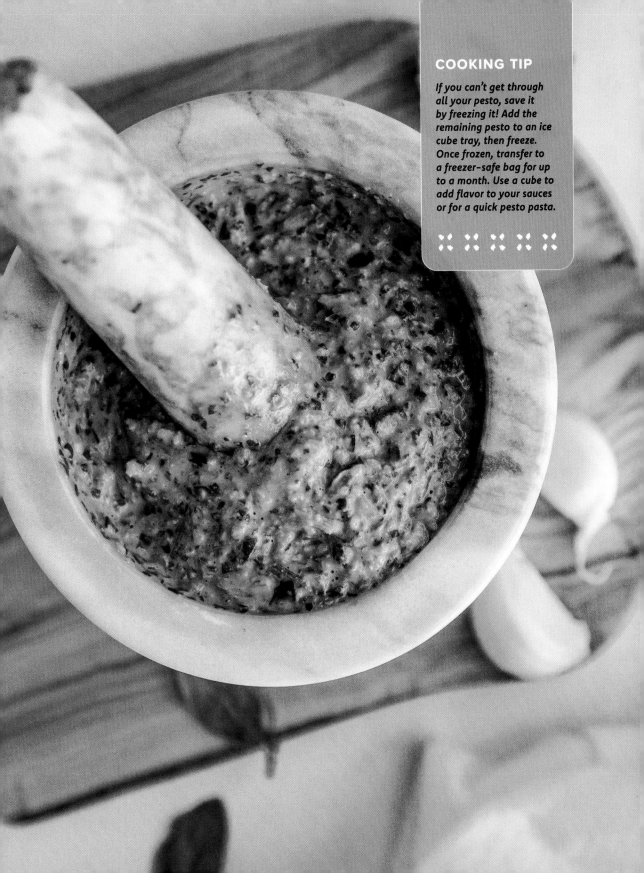

COOKING TIP

If you can't get through all your pesto, save it by freezing it! Add the remaining pesto to an ice cube tray, then freeze. Once frozen, transfer to a freezer-safe bag for up to a month. Use a cube to add flavor to your sauces or for a quick pesto pasta.

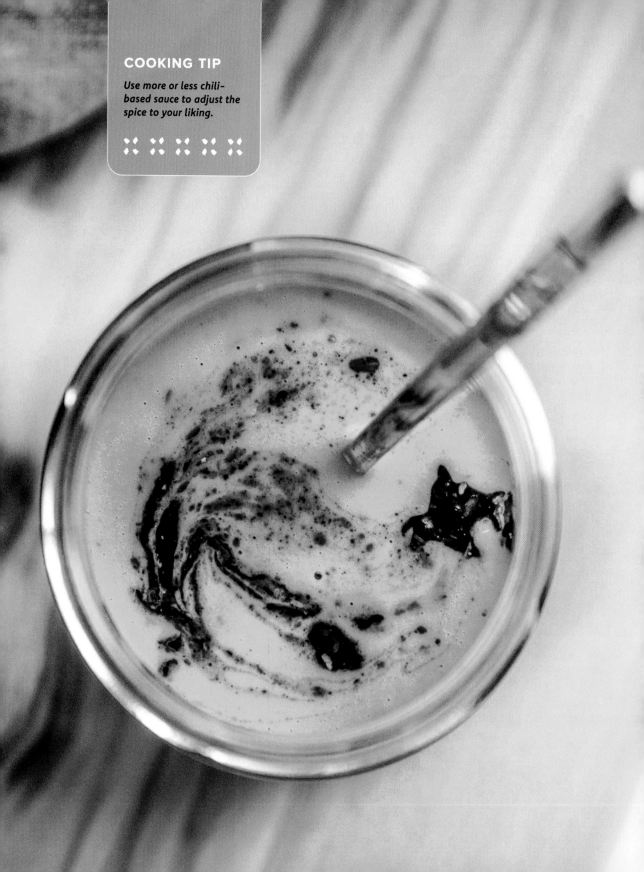

Peanut sauce is my go-to sauce because it's always so easy to put together. You just add every-thing to a bowl and whisk and it comes out so flavorful every single time. To make it even better, you can customize this one based on the amount of effort you want to exert. Now, I always try to encourage fresh ginger and garlic when possible because the flavors really do shine through. However, on those days you don't feel like grating or zesting, just measure out the recommended alternatives, and your sauce will still be super delicious.

Chili Crunch Peanut Sauce

MAKES ¾ CUP • PREP TIME: 5 MINUTES

3 tablespoons natural peanut butter

1 tablespoon tamari (see page xli)

1 tablespoon chili crisp oil or sriracha

2 teaspoons maple syrup

1 garlic clove, grated or ½ teaspoon garlic powder

½ teaspoon grated fresh ginger or ¼ teaspoon ground ginger

Zest and juice of 1 lime or 1 tablespoon rice vinegar

To a large glass measuring cup or bowl, add the peanut butter, tamari, chili crisp oil, maple syrup, garlic, ginger, and lime zest and juice. Whisk everything together and you will notice the sauce start to thicken.

Pour in 3 tablespoons water, then whisk again to thin out the sauce. If still too thick, add 1 tablespoon water at a time while whisking until your desired sauce consistency is achieved.

Transfer the sauce to an airtight container and store in the fridge for up to 7 days.

There are an incredible number of sauces from all around the world that are quick and simple to make no matter where you call home. One I've recently started incorporating into my weekly meal rotations is Zhoug (also written as *Zhug*). Zhoug is a style of hot sauce used in Yemeni cuisine. Now, preparation can vary household to household, but the main components typically include a combination of hot chili peppers, garlic, cumin, coriander, cilantro, and oil. Use this mostly as a guideline and modify the amount of spices, lemon, heat, or oil based on your own personal preference. Then use it to top your favorite recipes for a little extra heat and freshness.

Zhoug

MAKES 1 ¼ CUPS • PREP TIME: 15 MINUTES • COOKING TIME: 2 MINUTES

½ teaspoon cumin seeds

½ teaspoon coriander seeds

2 garlic cloves

½ teaspoon ground cardamom

1 cup packed fresh cilantro, woody stems removed

Juice of ½ lemon

2 serrano peppers, stems removed

½ teaspoon kosher salt, plus more to taste

¼ cup extra-virgin olive oil

Heat a small sauté pan over medium-low heat. Once hot, add the cumin seeds and coriander seeds. Stir the seeds to toast for about 1 minute or until they become slightly fragrant.

Transfer the seeds to a mortar and pestle with the garlic and crush them to form a paste.

Add the paste to a food processor with the cardamom, cilantro, lemon juice, serrano peppers, and salt and process until the mixture is all mixed together and very finely chopped.

While the food processor is still running, slowly pour in the olive oil. Once added, continue processing, scraping down the sides as needed until the sauce is mostly smooth.

Taste and adjust salt to preference, then transfer to an airtight container and allow to refrigerate for at least 1 hour before enjoying. This sauce can be stored in the fridge for up to 7 days.

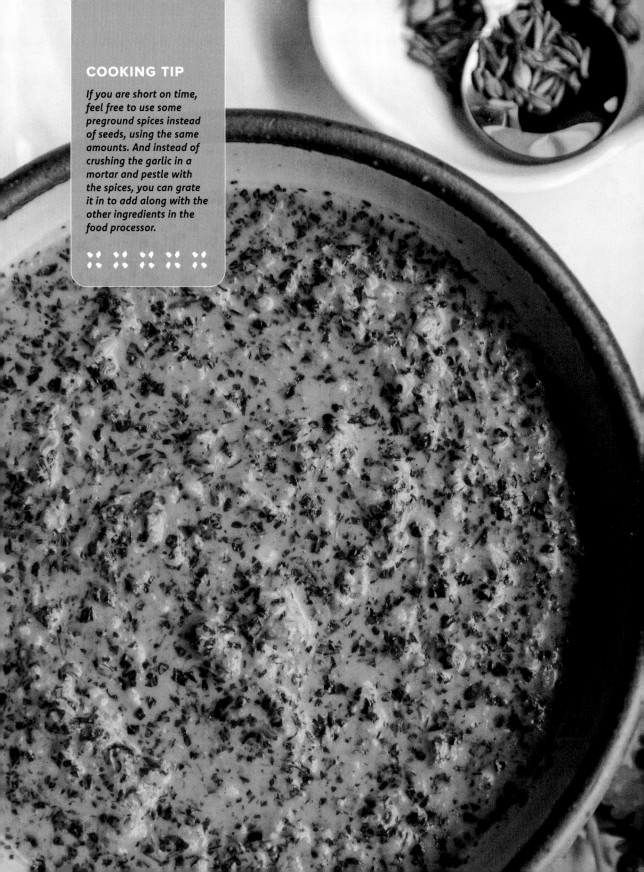

COOKING TIP

If you are short on time, feel free to use some preground spices instead of seeds, using the same amounts. And instead of crushing the garlic in a mortar and pestle with the spices, you can grate it in to add along with the other ingredients in the food processor.

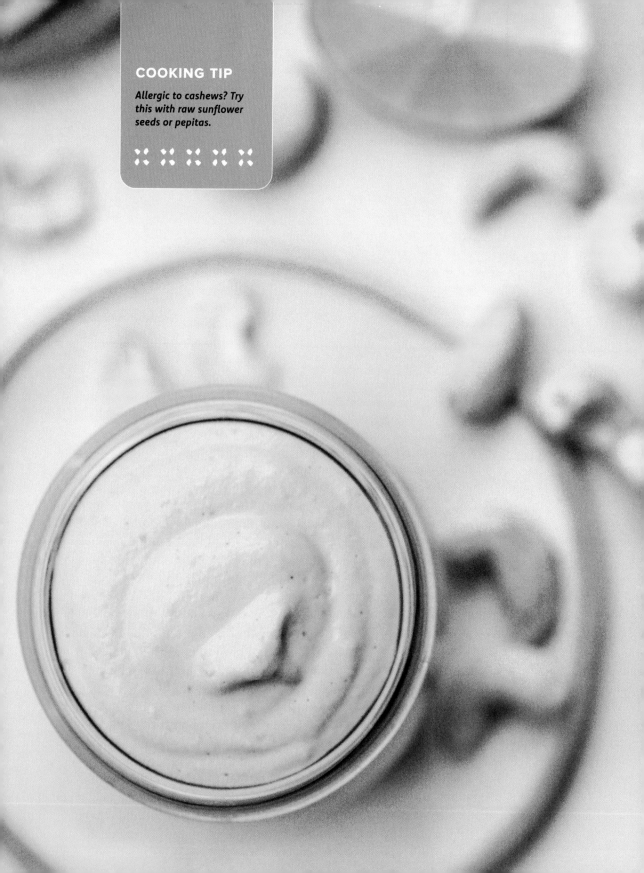

COOKING TIP

Allergic to cashews? Try this with raw sunflower seeds or pepitas.

I couldn't leave out crema, and this one just takes the basic traditional recipe and adds a punch of flavor that will keep you coming back for more. Since we are using cashews instead of dairy, we are adding a bunch of nutrition to this humble recipe. Cashews are rich in fiber, heart-healthy fats, and protein. They are also a good source of magnesium, which may support bone health. So if you like traditional crema, but are looking for a bump in nutrition, definitely give this one a try!

Jalapeño Lime Crema

MAKES 1 1/2 CUPS • PREP TIME: 20 MINUTES

1 cup raw cashews

2 cups boiling water, plus more as needed

1 jalapeño, stem removed and roughly chopped (for less spice remove seeds)

2 tablespoons nutritional yeast

Zest and juice of 1 lime

1/2 teaspoon garlic powder

1/2 teaspoon kosher salt, plus more to taste

Place the cashews in a heat-safe bowl. Add the boiling water to completely cover the cashews and allow to soften for 30 minutes.

Drain the cashews, then place in a blender with 1/2 cup fresh water, jalapeño, nutritional yeast, lime zest and juice, garlic powder, and salt. Blend until smooth.

Taste and adjust salt to preference and enjoy.

This is the sauce I make most. I call it Everything Sauce because I put it on everything—it's as simple as that! You just throw everything in a food processor and blitz it up, and it's ready to go. Make it at the start of the week to help make building nourishing meals a lot easier.

Everything Sauce

MAKES 1 ¼ CUPS • PREP TIME: 10 MINUTES

¼ cup packed fresh cilantro, stems removed

¼ cup packed fresh parsley, stems removed

1 garlic clove, grated or pressed

1 teaspoon red wine vinegar

½ cup plain unsweetened plant-based yogurt

1 teaspoon oregano

½ avocado

Zest and juice of 1 lemon

½ teaspoon kosher salt

Place the cilantro, parsley, garlic, vinegar, yogurt, oregano, avocado, lemon zest and juice, and salt into a food processor, then process on high until mostly smooth, which should leave the cilantro and parsley mostly minced in the sauce.

Taste and adjust salt to preference, then transfer the sauce into an airtight container and store in the fridge for up to 4 days. Use it to pair with tacos, to drizzle over your favorite bowls, or as a veggie dip!

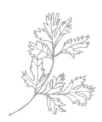

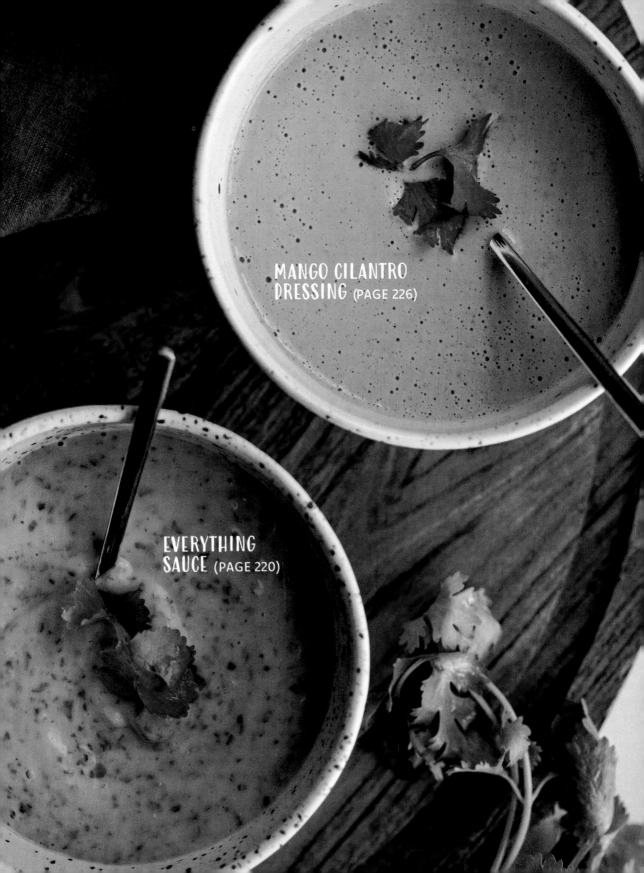

MANGO CILANTRO
DRESSING (PAGE 226)

EVERYTHING
SAUCE (PAGE 220)

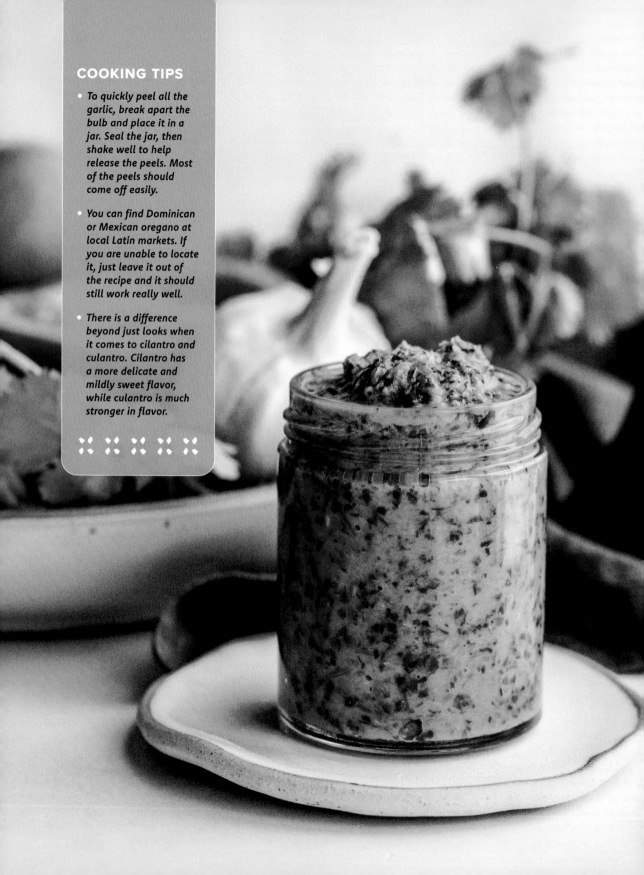

COOKING TIPS

- *To quickly peel all the garlic, break apart the bulb and place it in a jar. Seal the jar, then shake well to help release the peels. Most of the peels should come off easily.*

- *You can find Dominican or Mexican oregano at local Latin markets. If you are unable to locate it, just leave it out of the recipe and it should still work really well.*

- *There is a difference beyond just looks when it comes to cilantro and culantro. Cilantro has a more delicate and mildly sweet flavor, while culantro is much stronger in flavor.*

When my family would leave my Tio's house in Manhattan, he would send us away with bags of large plantains, salchichón, and an unmarked container of sazón (or sometimes it was stored in an empty tub of Country Crock, which was always a surprise when you were trying to butter your toast in the morning).

Sazón is a Dominican style sofrito, and every Dominican home I know makes theirs differently because we all have our own specific preferences. And even my own recipe has changed a lot based on ingredients I do or don't have access to. Regardless, having a blend of herbs, garlic, and onions together in the fridge will always add more rich flavor to your food. And this sofrito is intended for exactly that! Think of it like a flavor shortcut. Make a large batch, store it fresh or save in the freezer, and when you want to flavor your beans or stew, or even make a fantastic marinade, this sofrito will be waiting for you to use up.

Dominican Sofrito

MAKES 2 ¾ CUPS • PREP TIME: 15 MINUTES

2 garlic heads, peeled (about 26 cloves)

3 scallions, roots removed and roughly chopped

1 medium red onion, roughly chopped

1 cubanelle pepper or ½ green bell pepper

Kosher salt to taste

1 cup packed fresh cilantro leaves

½ cup packed fresh culantro (or more cilantro)

1 tablespoon apple cider vinegar

Juice of 1 lime

1 vegetable bouillon cube or 1 teaspoon vegetable bouillon paste

1 tablespoon Dominican oregano or Mexican oregano

2 tablespoons extra-virgin olive oil

To a food processor or blender, add the garlic, scallions, onion, pepper, and a generous pinch of kosher salt. Process on high until the ingredients are finely minced, stopping and scraping down the sides as needed.

Add in the cilantro, culantro, vinegar, lime juice, bouillon cube, oregano, and another pinch of salt, then blend again until it becomes a coarse paste.

Remove the blade of the food processor and stir in the oil.

You can store this in the fridge in an airtight container for up to 7 days. To preserve it even longer, freeze it! Divide the paste in an ice cube tray. Cover and freeze, then transfer the cubes into a freezer-safe bag or container and store in the freezer for up to 6 months. Use the cubes to add to your beans, stews, or marinades as a shortcut for extra flavor.

Yes, you can buy jam from the store, but you can also make a delicious homemade one with just five ingredients. Now, this one is special because we are using chia seeds to help thicken the jam. The benefit, an extra boost of omega-3s every time you spread this delicious jam on your morning toast.

Lemon Blueberry Chia Jam

MAKES 1 CUP • PREP TIME: 10 MINUTES • COOKING TIME: 7 MINUTES

2 cups frozen blueberries
(this works with other
berries, too)

2 tablespoons maple syrup

1 teaspoon vanilla extract

2 tablespoons chia seeds

Zest of 1 lemon

Place a medium saucepan over medium-low heat. Add the berries, maple syrup, and vanilla and allow the berries to cook and thaw for about 5 to 6 minutes.

Once thawed, use a potato masher or the back of your cooking spoon to gently mash the berries. Remove from the heat, then add the chia seeds and lemon zest and stir well to combine.

Allow to sit for 10 minutes, then stir well again. Transfer the berries to an airtight container and allow to cool completely before placing in the fridge to set and chill for at least 1 hour before using.

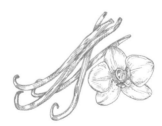

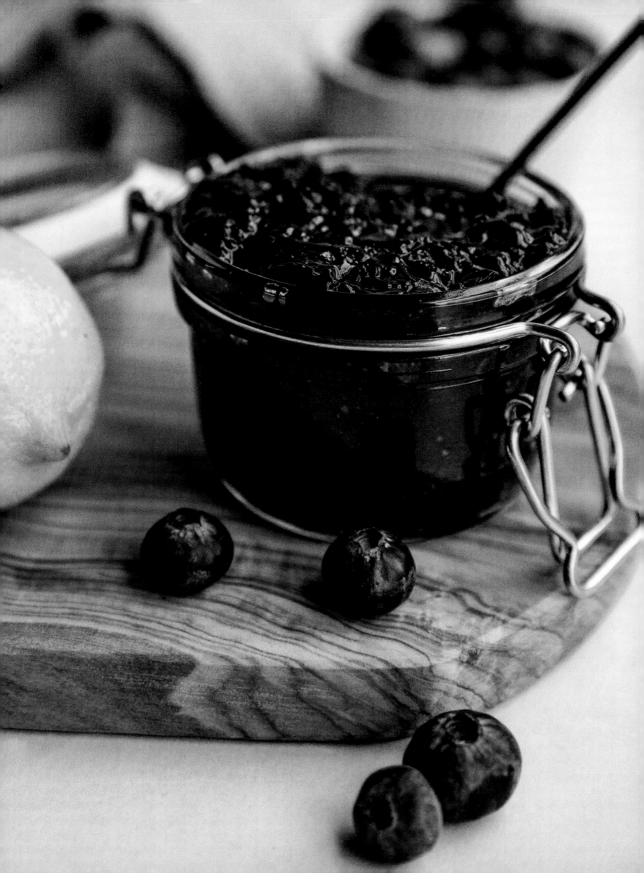

Make this the next time you have a ripe mango. This sauce is divine and has the perfect sweet tang that pairs well with salads, tacos, and your favorite nourishing bowls.

Mango Cilantro Dressing

MAKES 1 ¼ CUP • PREP TIME: 10 MINUTES

⅓ cup packed fresh cilantro leaves

½ cup mango, cubed (preferably Kent or Ataulfo mango)

½ cup plain unsweetened plant-based yogurt

Zest and juice of 1 lime

1 jalapeño, stem removed, roughly chopped

2 garlic cloves

2 tablespoons extra-virgin olive oil

¼ teaspoon kosher salt

Place the cilantro, mango, yogurt, lime zest and juice, jalapeño, garlic, oil, and salt into a blender cup and blend on high until completely smooth.

Pour the dressing into an airtight container then store in the fridge for up to 7 days.

COOKING TIPS

If you want your dressing to be less spicy, you can remove the seeds and veins of the jalapeño. Alternatively, you can also leave the pepper out entirely.

If you are familiar with mangoes, you might be less familiar with the fact that there are so many different types of mangoes available throughout the world. Typically, the most common varieties you see in the U.S. at local markets are Tommy Atkins, Kent mangoes, red mangoes, keitt mangoes, champagne or Ataulfo mangoes, and honey mangoes. Most often, the big difference between a lot of these varieties is the shape, color, and consistency of the flesh. The inside flesh of Tommy Atkins and red mangoes tends to be more fibrous in consistency whereas varieties like Kent and Ataulfo mangoes tend to have a softer, more buttery consistency, making them better for blending.

THE GRAINS AND LEGUMES COOKING GUIDE

After a lot of cooking, I've gotten to a point where batch-cooking grains and legumes at the start of the week is second nature. I've done it so much that I pretty much have this chart memorized and am confident with eyeballing things, too (my self-proclaimed superpower). Now I want you to feel just as confident. In the event you don't have a rice cooker or instant pot, these tips can help you successfully cook these items on the stovetop.

GRAINS OR LEGUMES (PER 1 CUP)	ADD THIS MUCH	COOKING TIME AND NOTES
Jasmine rice	1 cup plus 2 tablespoons water ½ teaspoon kosher salt	Rinse and drain the rice well. Place in a medium saucepan with water and salt. Bring to a boil, reduce to a low simmer, and cover. Cook for 12 to 13 minutes. Remove from heat and allow to stand 10 minutes covered to steam, then fluff with a rice paddle.
Short-grain brown rice	1¾ cup water 1 tablespoon soy sauce 2 dried shiitake mushrooms (optional)	Rinse and drain the rice well. Place in a medium saucepan with water, soy sauce, and mushrooms (if using). Bring to a boil, reduce to a low simmer, and cover. Cook for 40 minutes, remove from heat, and allow to stand 10 minutes covered to steam. Remove the mushrooms and fluff with a rice paddle.
Farro	Water Kosher salt	Fill a large saucepan with water and bring to a boil. Salt the water like you would for pasta. Add the farro and cook for 17 minutes. Drain, then place back in the pot without a lid for 5 to 10 minutes.
Quinoa	1¾ cup water or vegetable broth	Rinse the quinoa under cold water and drain well. Add to a pot with liquid and bring to a boil, then reduce to a simmer and cover. Cook 14 to 15 minutes, remove from heat, and let stand covered for 10 minutes, then fluff with a fork.
French lentils	3 cups vegetable broth 1 bay leaf	Rinse and drain the lentils. Place in a large saucepan with the vegetable broth and bay leaf and bring to a boil. Reduce to a simmer and cook covered for 15 to 17 minutes.
Chickpeas	Water 1 bay leaf 1 onion, quartered 8 garlic cloves, smashed	Soak the chickpeas overnight with enough water to cover the beans by 2 inches. Drain and rinse, then cover with 2 to 3 inches fresh water. Bring to a boil with the bay leaf, onion, and garlic, then simmer for 1½ to 2 hours. Toward the end of cooking, stir in salt to taste.

PUT IT ALL INTO PRACTICE

Now that you have all the information for balancing your meals, let's focus on balancing your day. Use the below template with the accompanying recipes as a way to mix and match the things you love while still staying in balance. All meal plan suggestions here follow the plant plate method, which means each plate contains a serving of starch, protein, and produce.

Please see individual recipe notes for tips about gluten-free ingredient alternatives. When swapping meal ideas, think of how you want to account for different plant-based categories to meet your specific nutrient needs. Lastly, to help with making meal planning easier, think about ways to save time using the tips from the meal prepping section (see page xliii).

Sample Meal Plan Day 1

BREAKFAST: Chocolate Chip Cookie Dough Oats (page 11)
served with ½ cup strawberries

LUNCH: High-Protein Red Lentil Falafel (page 140) served with warm pita bread,
fresh vegetables, and 2 to 3 tablespoons hummus

DINNER: Charred Scallion Pesto Baked Gnocchi (page 144)

SNACK: 1 Persian cucumber sliced into coins and served with 2 to 3 tablespoons hummus
mixed with 1 tablespoon Super Seed Mix (page 176)

Sample Meal Plan Day 2

BREAKFAST: Pesto "Egg" Salad Breakfast Toast (page 15) topped with ½ cup arugula

LUNCH: Pico de Gallo Bowl (page 81)

DINNER: 20-Minute Cilantro Lime Noodles (page 92)

SNACK: 1 serving unsweetened plant-based yogurt mixed with 1 to 2 teaspoons maple syrup and 1 tablespoon natural peanut butter, then topped with ½ cup raspberries and 1 tablespoon Super Seed Mix (page 176)

Sample Meal Plan Day 3

BREAKFAST: Breakfast Tostadas (page 23)

LUNCH: Sweet Sesame Udon Noodle Jar (page 76)

DINNER: Maple Dijon Roasted Carrots and Asparagus with Scallion Rice (page 101)

SNACK: 1 Wholesome Date and Pistachio Cookie (page 183)

Sample Meal Plan Day 4

BREAKFAST: Raspberry Matcha Chia Pudding (page 20)

LUNCH: High-protein lunch box using 2 High-Protein Onigiri (page 192), ½ cup Blistered Sesame Lime Edamame (page 195), sliced Persian cucumbers, and baby carrots

DINNER: Brothy Beans and Greens (page 111) served with 1 to 2 slices of toasted sourdough bread

SNACK: 2 Coconut Lime Energy Bites (page 179)

Sample Meal Plan Day 5

BREAKFAST: Sweet Potato Boats (page 19) with Smoky Maple Tempeh Hash (page 16) and sliced avocado

LUNCH: Peanut Miso Chickpea Salad Sandwich (page 64)

DINNER: Crispy Buffalo White Bean Tacos (page 128), served with Easy No-Mayo Slaw (page 157)

SNACK: 1 ounce whole grain or gluten-free crackers served with 1 tablespoon natural peanut butter or sunflower butter and 3 tablespoons Lemon Blueberry Chia Jam (page 224)

UNIVERSAL CONVERSION CHART

OVEN TEMPERATURE EQUIVALENTS

250°F = 120°C   400°F = 200°C

275°F = 135°C   425°F = 220°C

300°F = 150°C   450°F = 230°C

325°F = 160°C   475°F = 240°C

350°F = 180°C   500°F = 260°C

375°F = 190°C

MEASUREMENT EQUIVALENTS

Measurements should always be level unless directed otherwise.

⅛ teaspoon = 0.5 mL

¼ teaspoon = 1 mL

½ teaspoon = 2.5 mL

1 teaspoon = 5 mL

1 tablespoon = 3 teaspoons = ½ fluid ounce = 15 mL

2 tablespoons = ⅛ cup = 1 fluid ounce = 30 mL

4 tablespoons = ¼ cup = 2 fluid ounces = 60 mL

5 ⅓ tablespoons = ⅓ cup = 3 fluid ounces = 80 mL

8 tablespoons = ½ cup = 4 fluid ounces = 120 mL

10 ⅔ tablespoons = ⅔ cup = 5 fluid ounces = 160 mL

12 tablespoons = ¾ cup = 6 fluid ounces = 180 mL

16 tablespoons = 1 cup = 8 fluid ounces = 240 mL

INDEX

French lentils. *See* beans and lentils

frozen foods

    about, xxxvi, 3

    How to Make Frozen Veggies Taste Amazing, 168–69, *169*

fruits, xx–xxi, xxxv. *See also* individual fruits

G

garlic

    Garlic Yogurt Sauce, 54, *55*

    Roasted Garlic and Herb Tahini Dressing, 68, *208,* 211

ginger

    Braised Orange Ginger Brussels Sprouts, 154, *155*

    Orange Ginger Tahini Dressing, 48, *208,* 210

    Scallion Ginger Lentil Fried Rice, *104,* 105

    Sticky Ginger Tofu Meatballs, 122–24, *122*

Gnocchi, Charred Scallion Pesto Baked, 144–45, *146*

Gochujang Stir-Fried Green Beans, 150

Go-To High-Protein Red Lentil Curry, 85–87, *86*

grab it & go, 56–77

    Chopped Veggie Tzatziki Jar, 70–72, *70*

    Herby Cauliflower Stuffed Pita, 68–69, *69*

    Kale Caesar Salad Wrap, 58–60, *59*

    Kimchi Noodle Soup Jar, 66–67, *66*

    Peanut Miso Chickpea Salad Sandwich, 64, *65*

    Smoky Chipotle Tofu Wrap, 61–63, *62*

    Spicy Tunaless Salad Sandwich, 74–75, *74*

    Sweet Sesame Udon Noodle Jar, 76–77, *77*

grains, about, xxii–xxiii, 227–228

Green Beans, Gochujang Stir-Fried, 150

Grilled Lemongrass Seitan Skewers, 137–39, *138*

Grilled Maple Dijon Lettuce, 164–65, *165*

grocery essentials, xxxv–xlii

Guisado Marinade, Tofu, *119,* 120

H

Habichuelas Guisadas, 96–97, *97*

health, eating for. *See* plant-based cooking

herbs and spices, xxxvii–xxxviii. *See also* sauces

Herby Cauliflower Stuffed Pita, 68–69, *69*

High-Protein Onigiri, 192–93, *193*

High-Protein Red Lentil Falafel, 140–41, *141*

How to Make Frozen Veggies Taste Amazing, 168–69, *169*

Hummus Pasta, Baked, 90–91, *90*

I

iodine, xxviii

iron, xxvi

J

Jalapeño Lime Crema, 63, 128, 200, 218–19, *218*

Jalapeños, Easy Pickled, *170,* 171

Jam, Lemon Blueberry Chia, 8, 187, 224, *225*

K

kala namak, 14

kale

    in Brothy Beans and Greens, *110,* 111

    Creamy Lemon Miso Chopped Kale Salad, 44, *45*

    Kale Caesar Salad Wrap, 58–60, *59*

kimchi

    Kimchi Noodle Soup Jar, 66–67, *66*

    Smashed Cucumber Kimchi Edamame Salad, *42,* 43

L

legumes, 227–28. *See also* beans and lentils; chickpeas; peanuts and peanut butter

lemon

    Chocolate Lemon Mousse, 190–91, *190*

    Creamy Lemon Miso Chopped Kale Salad, 44, *45*

    Lemon Blueberry Chia Jam, 8, 187, 224, *225*

    Lemon Blueberry Swirl Loaf, 186–87, *186*

    Lemon Poppy Seed Overnight Oats, 8, *9*

    Seared Lemon Chickpea Salad, 40, *41*

    Sticky Lemon Tofu Marinade, 116, *118*

    Tomato Beans with Lemony Panko Crumbs, 106–7, *106*

Lemongrass Seitan Skewers, Grilled, 137–39, *138*

lentils. *See* beans and lentils

Lettuce, Grilled Maple Dijon, 164–65, *165*

ABOUT THE AUTHOR

CATHERINE PEREZ is a registered dietitian, nutritionist, and vegan plant-based-recipe developer with a passion for infusing both flavor and nutrition into balanced meals that aim to make you feel your best.

Catherine's food philosophy comes from a place of understanding that the world of nutrition and cooking can be intimidating for the average person. Avoiding the latest food that is being fearmongered online and knowing exactly what foods you should be aiming to include more of is stressful enough. Early on that same pressure around food didn't make the kitchen feel very peaceful to Catherine. However, after adopting a vegan diet and needing to gain a new understanding of cooking, she was able to heal her relationship with food, properly fuel herself using evidenced-based nutrition, and find solace in the kitchen. Now, with everything she has learned working with different clients throughout her dietetic career, she wants to bring that same feeling of peace to others and show them exactly how to apply the nutrition information she shares through nourishing meals.

So, wherever you are on your journey, Catherine is here to support you one step at a time and to help you eat more plants—and actually like them.

To learn more about Catherine visit her website at https://plantbasedrdblog.com/ and for more inspiration follow her on Instagram and TikTok: @plantbasedrd.

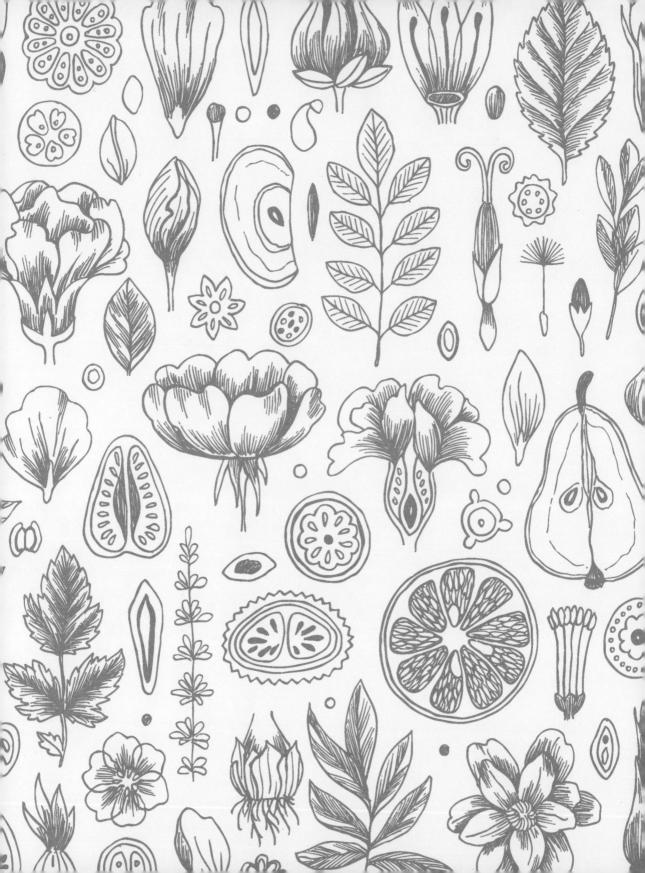